Lice Advice

The Shepherd Method™ of Strand by Strand Nit Removal

Katie Shepherd

Founder and CEO of The Shepherd Institute for Lice Solutions

StarGroup International Inc

DEDICATION

This book is dedicated to all the sweet innocent children
who have suffered through a case of head lice,
allowing me the hands-on experience
needed to make this book possible.

May you never itch again!

Ms. Katie

Published 2009

StarGroup International
West Palm Beach, Florida
561.547.0667
www.stargroupinternational.com

FIRST EDITION

Edited by Gwen Carden
Cover and book design by Mel Abfier
Cartoon illustrations by Terry Van Rhyn

Printed in Korea

LICE ADVICE - The Shepherd Method of Strand by Strand Nit Removal

ISBN 978-1-884886-92-8

Photos by Cyndi McCranie

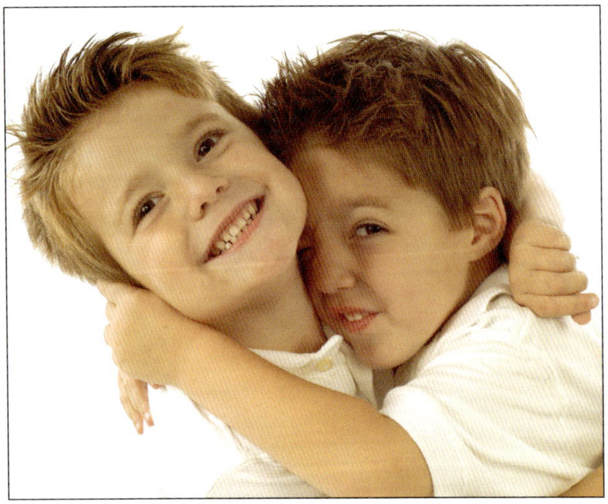

A portion of all profits will go to benefit lice treatment services for needy children.

This book is designed to provide information on a trademarked and field-tested, proprietary head lice treatment process. It is sold with the understanding that the publisher and author are not engaged in rendering medical advice or services. If medical care is needed, the services of an appropriately licensed health care professional should be sought.

This text should be used as a general guide. It is not meant to be a substitution for medical advice or care. The purpose of the text is meant to educate and also entertain.

The author and publisher shall have neither liability nor responsibility to any person or entity with respect to any loss or damage caused or alleged to have been caused, directly or indirectly, by the information contained in this book.

1 2 3 4 5 6 7 8

CONTENTS

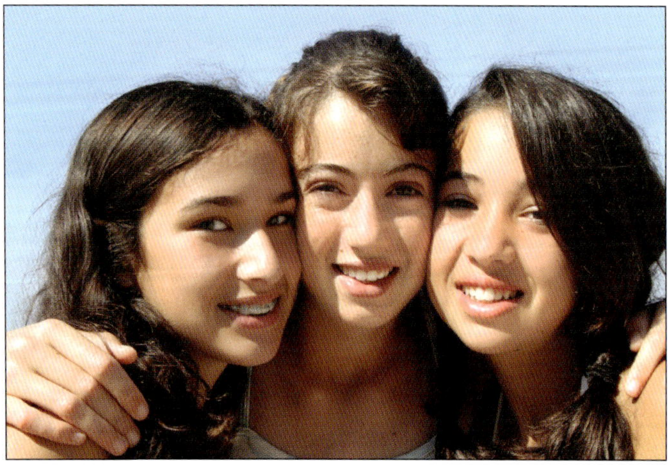

FOREWORD

Head lice, a highly stigmatized condition, affects people of all ages and walks of life. It is estimated that 6-12 million people in the United States will experience head lice each year. Despite the large number of people who experience head lice annually, members of the health care community often see head lice as a nuisance rather than as a problem that significantly impacts families. Many parents know the frustration of finding reliable information while trying to treat head lice on their own.

The primary mode of head lice transmission is head to head contact, making transmission between family members likely. Research studies addressing this condition are focused primarily on the efficacy of treatment products designed to kill head lice and their eggs (nits) and rarely focus on the spread of head lice within family settings.

The publication of Lice Advice: The Shepherd Method™ of Strand by Strand Nit Removal provides families with a powerful treatment weapon to use against head lice. The Shepherd Method™ was developed over the past 10 years and has been used to successfully treat thousands of children and adults. The book offers step-by-step instruction on techniques that provide caregivers with the tools they need to screen and treat all family members for head lice. Color photographs make the process come to life!

My research involving families with persistent head lice suggests there is significant psychological stress and caregiver strain involved in caring for family members with head lice and supports the need for improved family oriented educational materials. Lice Advice: The Shepherd Method™ of Strand by Strand Nit Removal is an important step toward providing access to safe, effective head lice treatment for all families.

Shirley C. Gordon, Ph.D.
Director, Florida Atlantic University
Head Lice Treatment and Prevention Project
Christine E. Lynn College of Nursing
Florida Atlantic University
sgordon@fau.edu

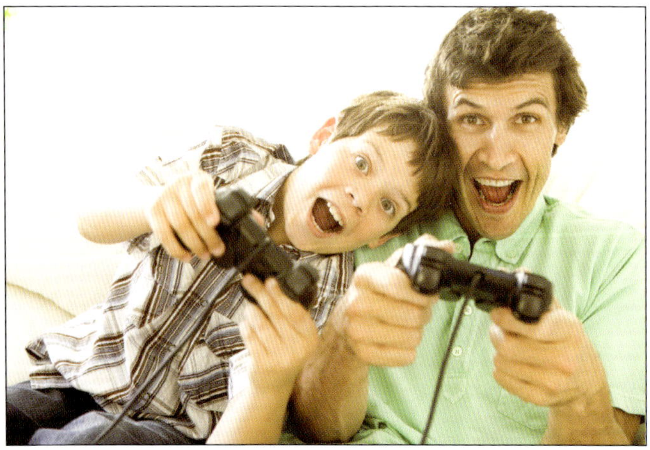

PREFACE

I'm writing in support of Katie Shepherd, who is an expert in human lice, their treatment and removal, and in the counseling of parents and children about head lice. I have known Katie for four years. In my research I study the evolutionary history of human lice (all of them) to infer evolutionary events in human history. For example, human head lice show the genetic signature of a population expansion 100,000 years ago, which coincides with modern human emergence out of Africa. Katie has helped tremendously with our research projects in many ways. Given the length of time that I have known her, and the close interactions we've had, I feel more than qualified to recommend her to you as an author for a book on head lice and their removal (which is sorely needed).

Katie has been at the forefront of her field for many years now, and has set up the preeminent model for louse-removal facilities. Katie has been a source of knowledge for my research group at the University of Florida for many years, and I go straight to her when I need the most up-to-date information about head lice.

Many "home remedies" exist for the treatment of head lice, and some are extremely dangerous yet often used (e.g., kerosene). Teaching families how to deal with the often-recurring problem of head lice appropriately is critical. Because of no-nit policies (children cannot return to school if nits, louse eggs, are visible) children miss school and parents miss work. Parents become panic stricken and utterly frustrated over lice and the difficulty of effectively removing them. And, because the lice are resistant to many insecticidal shampoos, populations are on the rise all over North America (and in developed countries worldwide).

Katie is among the leaders in the field of debunking myths and dangerous home remedies, and is incredibly well respected among her patients, colleagues, scholars, and peers. I can think of no one better suited for writing a book on head lice, especially one on nit and louse removal.

David L. Reed, Ph.D.

Florida Museum of Natural History
University of Florida

ACKNOWLEDGEMENTS

I have often wondered how any author could begin to name the vast number of people who in one way or another helped contribute to the completion of their book. This one was ten years in the making, and thus I have no doubt that that there will be some who have been left out in the acknowledgements below. To those people I extend my deepest apologies. While I have had years to contemplate what I wanted to convey within the pages of this book, the sudden urgency to meet a press deadline has not allowed me the same luxury of time to consider all those I would like to thank.

First and foremost I wish to thank my husband, Brad, and daughter Ashley. Without their patience and understanding, allowing me the time to return late night phone calls to desperate parents and spend hours in front of the computer answering e-mails, the experiences gained that helped lead to this book would not have been possible. Thanks especially to my husband Brad, what can I say? Few men would give up season tickets to their favorite college football team so that their wife could follow her dreams. From the start it was he who helped to pave the way. At his suggestion I started the first outreach program. His faith in me kept me going even when I became discouraged. Like myself, Brad believed there was more to be done in the fight against head lice.

I also want to thank Ashley, who has literally grown up with head lice as a dinner topic. I appreciate her willingness to stand tall and recognize that while head lice may not have been the coolest topic among her friends, it was a job that did make a difference. Seeing so many of her friends receive our services helped there as well.

I also wish to thank my son Jason for running deposits, picking up supplies for the office and tending to the many jobs that needed a man's touch. On behalf of my entire staff, I thank you.

I also extend thanks to my oldest son Chad for his loyal dedication to anything I needed done. By always looking out for each other we have helped nurture the best in each other. I want him to know how very proud I am of the man he has become and I thank him for allowing me to be the kind of mother he could be proud of as well.

To my daughter Tara I am grateful for her never-ending words of encouragement, for being a sounding board when I needed one and for helping out at so many fundraising events. Thanks also to the spouses of my eldest children: Kat for her early services as a lice technician and for always being the first to volunteer when I needed a helping hand. Thanks to Lumy for helping rebuild our website and overseeing so many of my computer needs. Thanks also for helping me make spreadsheet deadlines for critical presentations. Her wealth of knowledge and willingness to always step forward is more appreciated than she will ever know. Thanks to Kevin as well for helping with fundraising events and adding a little muscle when we needed it.

No acknowledgement would be complete without the mention of my sweet grandchildren. Rebecca, Chloe, Joseph, Beau and Luminosa, I love you dearly. Hopefully the efforts put forth over the last ten years will help to ensure you a lice-free future.

Few people are blessed with so many willing family members, and while I admit that I have taken advantage of their kindness, it was never without great appreciation. I thank my brother Ron for all his proofreading, even when I left him little time to accomplish it. Thanks for his advice and hands-on help and for being an early donor when we needed the financial help so much.

Thanks to my sister Cyndi for being a proud believer and for allowing us to use her kids (OK, so they had head lice) as early subjects, as we toiled to perfect our technique. I appreciate her being a voice in her community and for proudly promoting the efforts of our non-profit organization. Thanks also for her contribution to this book. Cyndi, a photographer for Disney, used her down time to help provide us with quality photos that have clearly illustrated for parents the steps necessary for treating their children. Her services and support are invaluable.

Thanks to my dad, Stan, also a photographer, for his assistance in filming fundraising events and photographing promotional material. What would I do without each and every one of them?

My bother-in-law Kevin, his wife, Michelle, and my sister-in-law Deborah, all willingly gave up many a 4th of July to help provide me with enough bodies to staff our event booth. It's reassuring that in times of need they truly were there for me. I owe you big time and I'm sure at least Kevin will remind me of it.

Thanks to my mother-in-law Pat, who has come to my rescue on many occasions and has willingly offered to help any way she could, including answering the phones.

I especially want to thank my mother Eleanor. While she might have doubted my early wisdom, she always stood by me. She has been my biggest fan, my strongest supporter, and though she reminds me regularly that I work too hard, she has always been there to help fuel my dreams. Without her allowing me to fall back on her in times of need, our non-profit agency might never have made it this far. I can't thank her enough for helping me fulfill my dreams. I love you, Mom!

What would any office be without dedicated staff? My West Palm Beach office manager Melinda Lopez has been with me since early on. One of my oldest and dearest employees, she has tirelessly helped build my staff and perfect our technique. Who knew when Melinda first entered our office seeking help for her own children that she would one day become such a vital part of our organization?

Thank you to our assistant manager Delmi Artiga for all her help. While she would rather have accompanied me on my many trips to New Hampshire, she willingly stepped in for Melinda, allowing her a much needed break. Hang in there Delmi, your turn is coming.

I wish to thank Abby Irwin, my office manager in Nashville. Also a past client, she has worked passionately to ensure that the services we provided her family remain available for others as well.

No lice treatment facility would be able to operate without the capable hands of hard-working technicians. Thanks to their loyal dedication and meticulous work in everything they do, countless families have been served. Thanks to Marisol Moreno, our lead technician, for her willingness to always go above and beyond the call of duty. Her kind and gracious manner humbles me. To Viola Rangel for her attention to detail no matter what task she is handed. Her efforts on my behalf, have made my job much easier. I'm grateful to Sandy Moreno, whose bubbly personality is contagious and who is willing to help wherever needed, including traveling to other states. Then there's Claudia Marin who makes me look good with her talent for decorating and willingness to take over the role of the office's party organizer. Brandy Rosenbeck, a kind and gentle heart if there ever was one, is the best when it comes to calming young children, who naturally gravitate to her. Thanks to Robin Burkett for being Abby's right hand and for always being available, even at the last minute. Few people possess the congenial personality of Rana Lattimore. Although we hired her as a lice technician, a role at which she has excelled, she is so much more than that to our organization. Thanks also to our computer guru, Chris Beckstrom. He has kept our computers going, allowing us the opportunity to work nonstop on this book. I especially appreciate his making it possible for families to order the book online at www.liceadvicebook.com (and putting this site up on such short notice). Thanks to my front office for taking so much burden off my shoulders/to Peter Goodge for so passionately helping parents in need, and to Kathleen McManus for having some of the fastest typing fingers in Palm Beach County. If not for Kathleen's ability to decipher my sloppy handwriting and the speed within which she turned the pages around, this book would have taken even more years to get into print.

While some may refer to them as my staff, I call them my right and left arms. If not for the ongoing support and encouragement of my Administrative Director, Gina Pierce, and my Director of Research Projects, Rossmeri Montalvo, this book would still be nothing more than a dream. When I hired Gina, I knew that she possessed awesome organizational skills, as well as the ability to motivate people. In the short time that she has been with our organization, she's been responsible for the completion of countless projects. Realizing that what I desired most was a clone of myself, she has worked nonstop to prove that she could be that - and a whole lot more. It didn't take me long to realize that Rossmeri and I possessed some of the same entrepreneurial qualities. Both fueled by a good challenge, we have worked aggressively to move Lice Solutions to a level that ensures a secure and prosperous future for our organization. Bringing this book to fruition on such a short deadline was no easy challenge. However like me, Gina and Rose are workaholics who ensure that one way or another, deadlines are met. They love their job and take satisfaction in knowing that they are making a difference. Although they are proud of what we've achieved so far, it is only the beginning. Watch out world, here they come! Gina and Rose you're more than co-workers - you're the best of friends. I love you both.

I decided a few of years ago that the best way to reach the countless households that lacked the kind of services offered in our community was to write a book. While it was a great plan and one that I immediately began by formulating an inital outline, my lack of time prevented me from moving it forward. If not for the encouragement of Dr. Shirley Gordon, Director of Head Lice Treatment and Prevention Projects with the Christine E. Lynn College of Nursing at Florida Atlantic University, this project would still be in the planning stages. Dr. Gordon and I have assisted each other in many ways. Each passionate about helping children, we have mutually sought ways to better educate the families we serve. Our ongoing collaborations predate even Melinda, and through it all we have grown to respect each other not only professionally but also as friends. Thanks, Shirley, for your devotion to both the fight against head lice and my need to do something about it.

I'd like to thank Kelly Addison for banding parents together to form PAHLS (Parents Advocating Head Lice Solutions) and for refusing to allow her community to ignore proactive head lice measures. Thanks as well to Jeff Hester who started out as a business associate but is now a wonderful friend and campaigner for what is right when it comes to helping families with head lice. Thanks to Dr. Harold Bafitis for introducing us to our publisher and therefore making this opportunity possible, and Cheryl McCarthy for believing in the parent's need for updated information and for continually encouraging me to get that information out there. Thanks also to the many volunteers who have helped throughout the years and to those individuals who have kindly donated to Lice Solutions, ensuring services for thousands of children. Thanks to the clients who have used our services and referred others to us. While we hope you never need us again, we are here for you if you do.

Finally, thanks to all those at Star Group International, and especially to my publisher Brenda Star, for believing in this book and helping transform my dream into a reality, far better than anything I had envisioned. Thanks to their Creative Director Mel Abfier for so patiently guiding us, allowing the manuscript to evolve into a book we could be proud of. Last but not least, thank you to Gwen Carden for the many hours she spent editing and proofreading the manuscript. It couldn't have been an easy task reading about head lice. Although I am aware that it left her itching for alternative reading, I can't thank her enough for all her help.

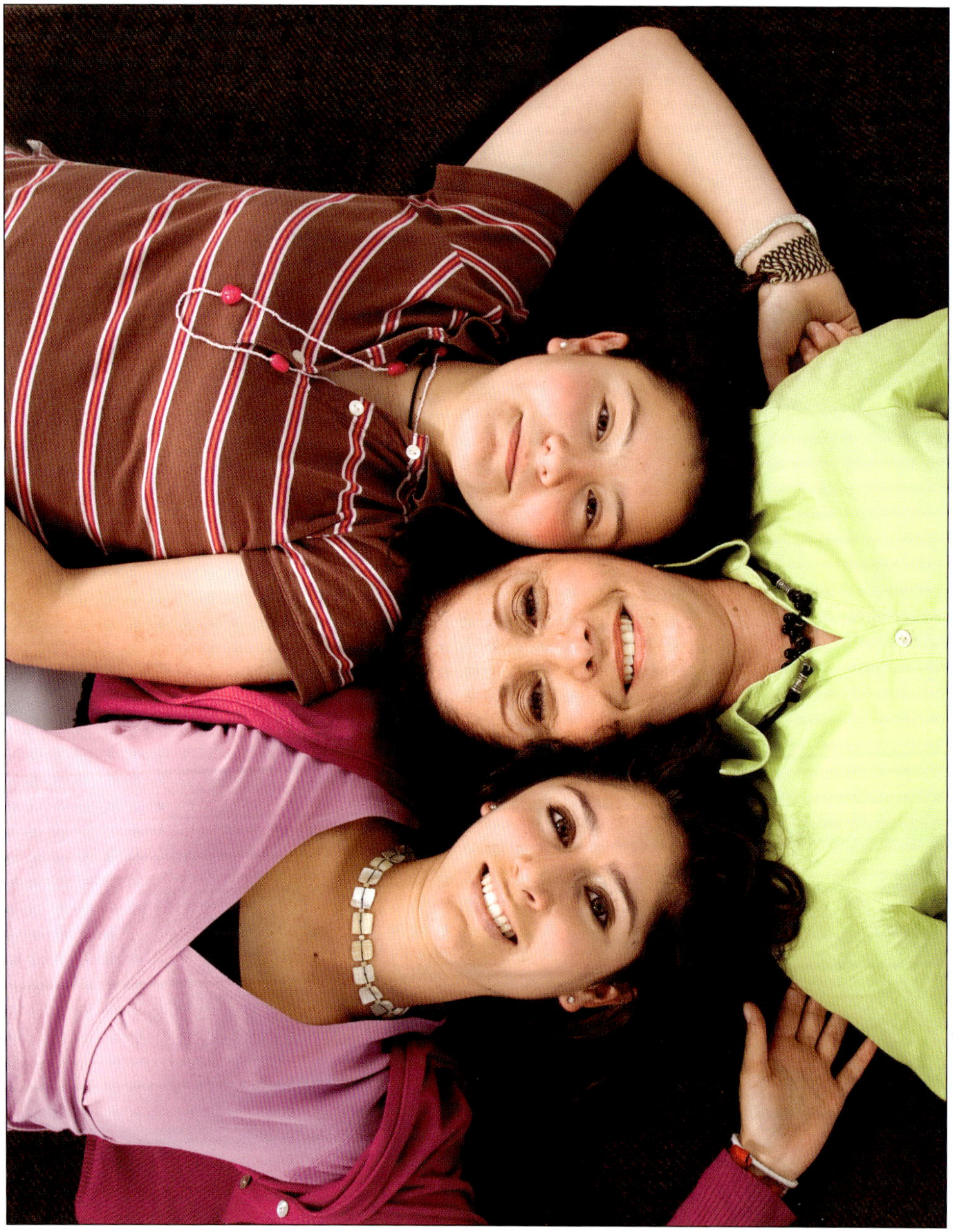

INTRODUCTION

I can hear it now: "***Head lice, yuck! Why would anyone want to read about head lice?***" Unless you have had the misfortune of dealing with head lice it's hard to appreciate the need for the information found in this book. However, if you are a parent who discovers this unwanted houseguest in your home, you'll quickly develop an unquenchable thirst for any information related to head lice that you can find. When parents enter our office they tell of countless nights of desperately trying to get rid of the tiny parasites and untold hours scouring the internet; frantically trying to learn everything they can about head lice in a frustrated attempt to put an end to this nightmare.

Head lice are not your mother's bugs! That's right - head lice as we know them today have changed. They have evolved into a newer and stronger breed that no matter what you do, you can't seem to get rid of them. After years of constant exposure to pesticides, the bugs have built up resistance to some of the very products developed to eliminate them, leaving many people feeling discouraged and all alone. As if that isn't bad enough, much of the available information is so outdated that it sends families in circles, resulting in wasted hours on things that make little difference. As we tell our parents every day, "*The internet is a wonderful tool. It provides a wealth of information at our fingertips. However, it is also a source for recycling old, outdated information.*" Sadly even the media, as well as many well-intended medical experts, rely on these resources for their facts, thus breathing new life into this wealth of misinformation.

Parents regularly comment "*I've cleaned everything. I threw away all the pillows. I wash the sheets every day. The toys have been bagged for the past month, but no matter what I do I just can't seem to get rid of the lice. What am I doing wrong*?" These parents, like so many others, are spending too much time focusing on all the wrong things and not enough time on the things that really matter. Unfortunately, head lice is *the gift that keeps on giving*! Imagine setting up a chain of dominoes and then tapping the first one. As we all know, that first domino sets off a chain reaction that just continues going and going, or in the case of head lice, giving and giving! It is possible to put an end to your part of the chain, by stopping the spread and ending the cycle that allows them to come back at you again. To do that, however, we must recognize and deal with the true problem.

A past client once told me that when she mentioned our facility to her pediatrician, hoping the doctor might be willing to refer others in need of our service, the doctor casually remarked, "*A place that treats head lice? Please! I can tell you everything you need to know about head lice on one sheet of paper.*" The parent, having already been sold on the benefits of the kind of hands-on help we offer, told the doctor "*I guess that tells me what you don't know about head lice*!"

Many doctors are the first to admit that they don't know nor want to know, anything about head lice. Just as many pediatricians in our area are thankful for the services we provide and tell us, "W*hen a patient calls our office and mentions lice, we tell them DO NOT bring them into the office. We quickly give them your phone number.*" A large percentage of our referrals come from medical practitioners who have brought their own children to us for treatment. They recognize the importance of eliminating the problem quickly. The one thing medical professionals who appreciate the lice problem all seem to agree on is that the prescription products currently on the market are NOT an option for their children.

It is my hope to better educate you with updated head lice information by sharing the knowledge gained from years of service, clinical research and client experiences and in doing so spare you wasted time, money and needless product exposure. If we can prevent just one parent from resorting to dangerous treatment options or drastic measures that often affect the child's self esteem, this book will have served its purpose.

Forget everything you thought you knew about head lice. *Lice Advice* shares what works and what doesn't through newer research and years of hands-on experience.

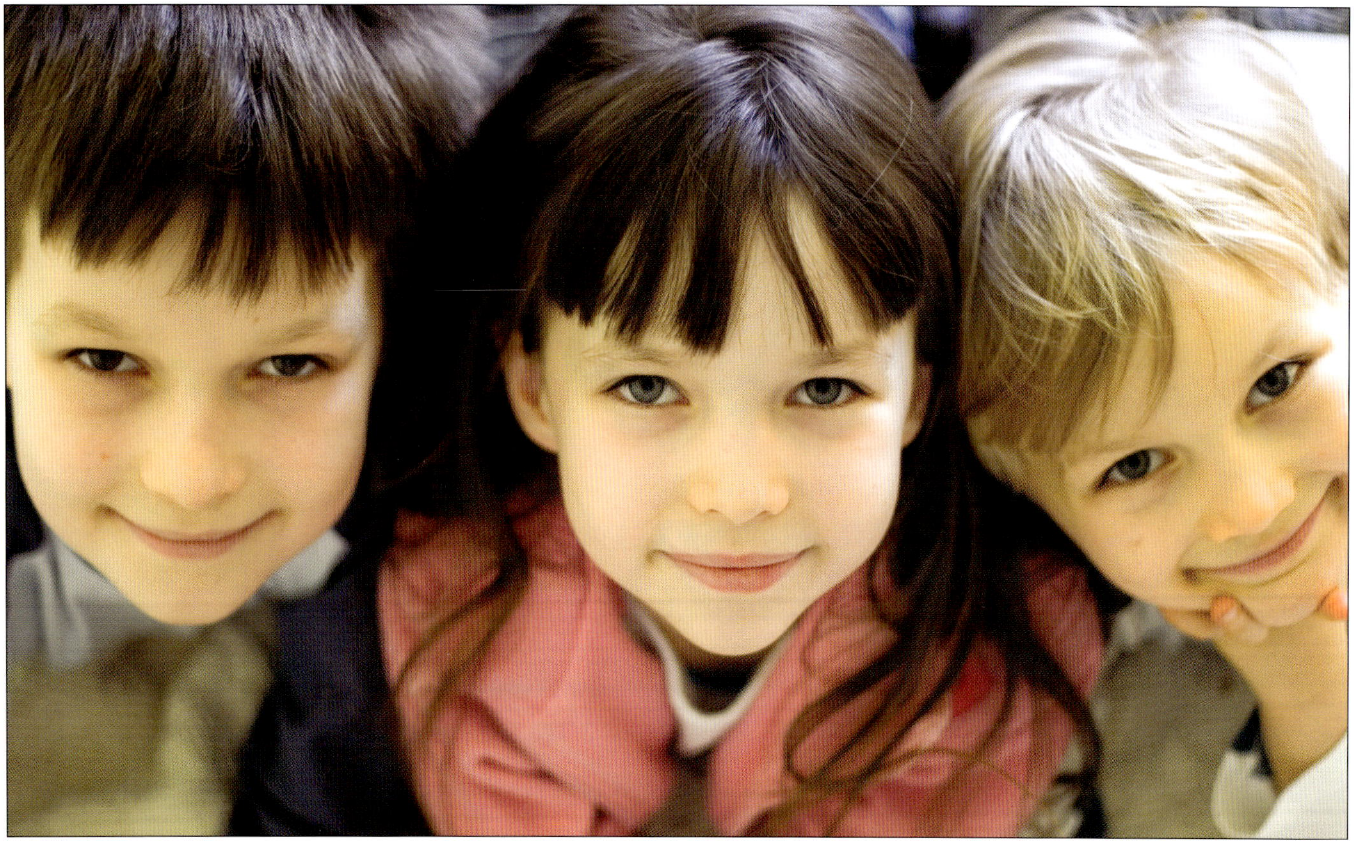

1

FACTS OF LICE

Understanding the problem helps bring about solutions. ***Lice Solutions!***

What are head lice?
Where do they come from?
How do we get them?
Why me?
Do only children get head lice?
Aren't lice a sign of being dirty?
Will it help if I wash my child's hair daily?
What about putting lots of gel on my child's hair?
How do I know for sure that my child has head lice?
What if I find head lice?
How bad is the problem?
Why has it become such a problem?
Is there any danger?
What is being done about it?
How can I help?

"You'll notice that some words are in **bold** lettering. Any word that is printed in **bold** letters is a definition word regarding "The *Shepherd* Method™."

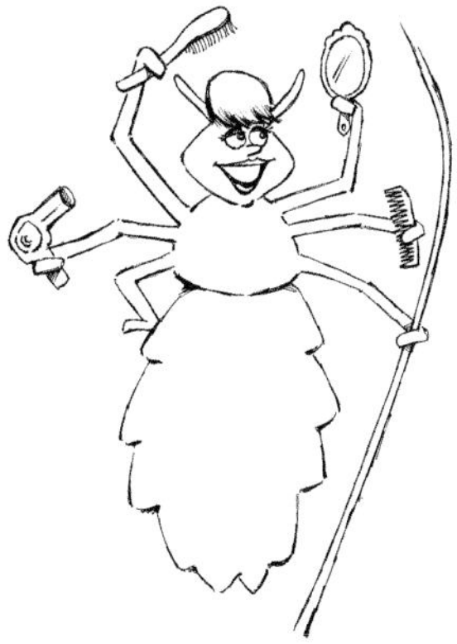

What are head lice?

Head lice are tiny, six-legged, blood-sucking parasites. Each leg is equipped with a claw, enabling the louse to grasp onto the shaft of the hair. They range in size from 2mm to 4mm, approximately the size of a sesame seed. Females are generally longer and wider than males and have a more rounded stomach. Male lice, unlike their female counterparts, have a brown band across their backs. They can vary in color from grayish white to reddish brown. Head lice, like chameleons, have the ability to adapt to their environment. Head lice found on dark-haired or dark-skinned individuals will most likely be darker than those found on blond-haired or lighter-skinned individuals. Other factors that can affect the color of the louse are environmental temperature, sunlight, even blood intake. A louse will appear darker in warm temperatures or bright lights than those found in cooler climates. Additionally, a louse with a full stomach may also appear darker than its hungry counterpart. In some cases a louse will have a bright red appearance, especially if it has recently fed.

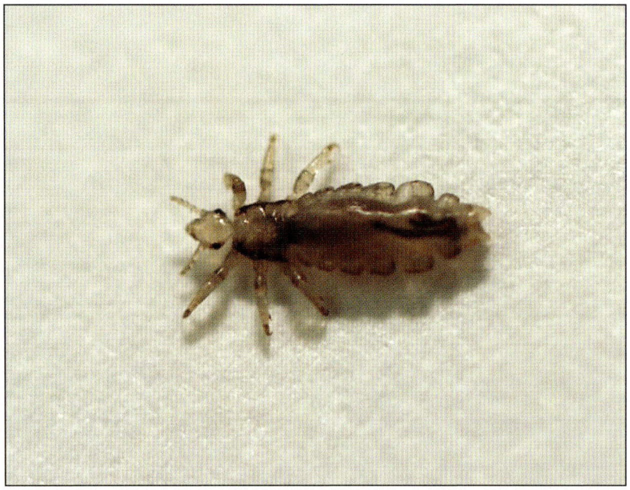

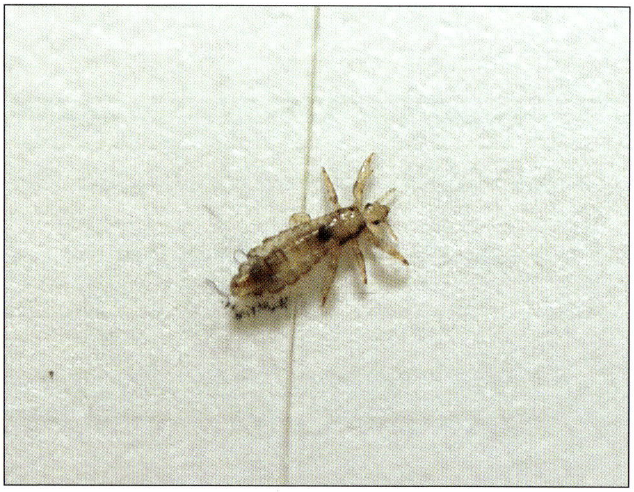

Pictured on the left – adult female louse; on the right – adult male louse. Note that the female is wider than the male and that her body ends in a "V" shape, while the male's body is narrower with horizontal stripes along the back. His body ends in a rounded point.

The female louse lays eggs by gluing them to the hair shaft. This glue is so fast-drying that in some instances the louse glues herself to the hair. She lays twice a day and can lay as many as five eggs at a time - a production rate that will generate some 200 eggs in her lifetime. Eggs, or nits as they're commonly called, generally hatch in seven to ten days. Newly hatched nymphs take another seven to ten days to reach adulthood. Once hatched, they have a life expectancy of approximately 30 days.

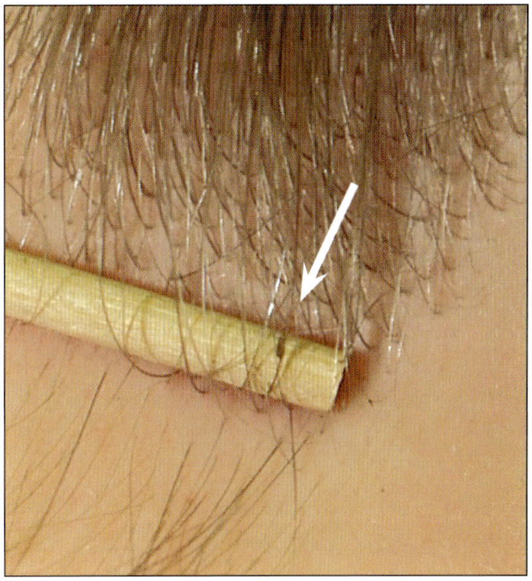

Pictured here is a nit on the hair. Nits blend with hairs and can be hard to identify, especially for the untrained individual.

Lice do not have jointed bodies, hind legs or wings. It is anatomically impossible for them to jump or fly. They can, however, move with amazing speed. An adult louse can travel as fast as nine inches per minute. An antenna located in front of the eyes enables the louse to detect odor, humidity, temperature and, it's believed, even blood types, in an attempt to identify a favorable source of blood. When head lice find a desirable environment they literally run to the new host. They have strong survival instincts and run to avoid exposure to bright lights or offensive odors. While they move quickly towards a favorable environment, they move just as quickly to avoid an undesirable one.

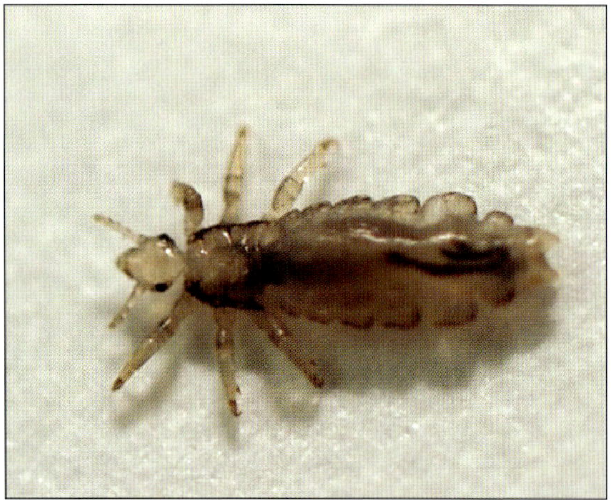

Note the antenna located in front of the eyes. These help the louse detect their food source.

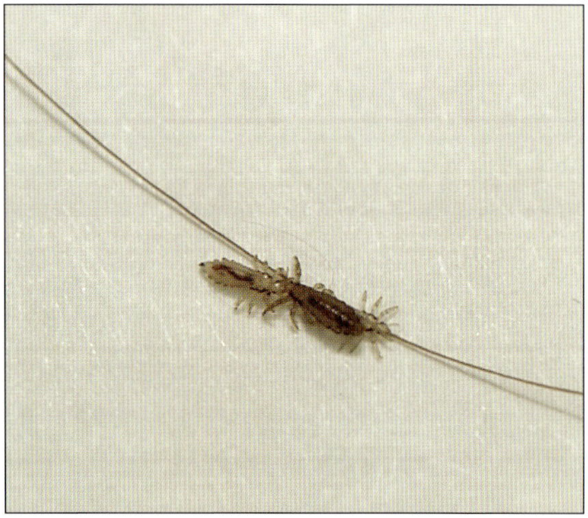

It's not uncommon to find several lice in one area. Look closely at the picture and see how many lice you find?

The answer is 3.

Head lice depend on human blood for survival. A louse separated from its human host will rarely survive more than 24 hours. Research has revealed that while head lice can survive for up to 24 hours off the human head, after approximately ten to twelve hours the bugs become dehydrated. Even if the lice were to find their way onto a new host at this point they would die because they are too weak to secrete saliva, which they must do to feed. Eggs found on an abandoned strand of hair have an even lower chance of survival as they would have to hatch within the first 24 hours or they will not hatch. Eggs need the warmth of the body to incubate, much like a chicken sitting on an egg. To survive off the head would require the egg to be close to hatching, similar to a fetus who is nine months old compared to two months old. Once hatched, nymphs, as "newborn" lice are called, must feed within the first two hours, as they require immediate feeding for survival. Like any newly hatched creature, they are not very agile. For a newly hatched nymph to find its way to your head requires that your head be at the exact spot in the exact moment that the egg hatches! Recognizing these facts allows us to better understand why the environment is not as big an issue as once thought. The real problem is the lice that remain on the head and the heads of those around us.

Where do they come from?

No one knows for sure, but evidence of lice goes back many centuries. Their shells have been found on mummies once sealed in ancient tombs, as well as in prehistoric burial grounds in North America. There are literary references to lice as far back as 16 B.C., where Egyptians once concocted their own remedies for head lice.

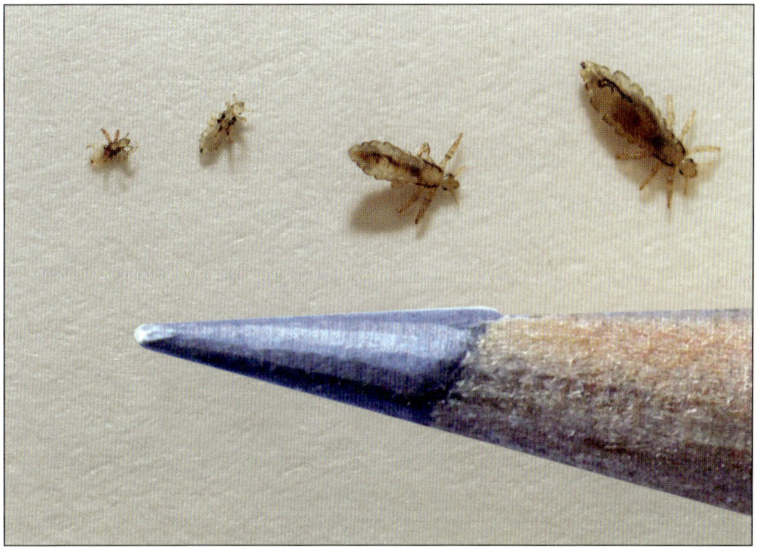

Pictured above from left to right; 1st stage nymph (just hatched), 2nd stage nymph, 3rd stage nymph, adult louse. Note the size of each in comparison to a very sharp #2 pencil.

George Washington spoke of head lice when, at age 13, he wrote a book on manners stating: "It's not polite to pick your lice in public, but if you see a louse on the head of a friend, it is polite to pick theirs."

How do we get them?

In most cases head lice are transmitted from one human to another, primarily through head-to-head contact. While most references report them as most commonly found on children ranging from ages three to eleven, newer research shows the largest number of cases are found in children between the ages of nine and 16.

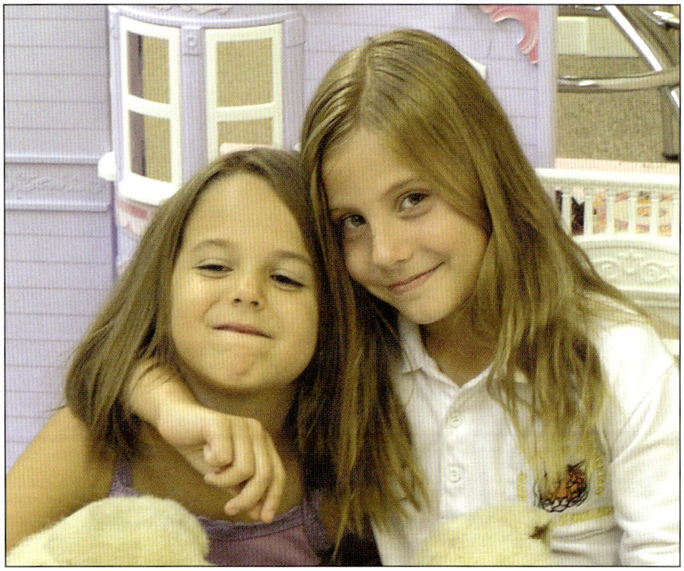

Head-to-head contact is the most common way to transmit head lice.

While it is possible to pick up a hitchhiker (an abandoned strand of hair with a louse still attached), it is suspected that less than 2% of all active cases are actually contracted in this manner. Lice eggs, or nits as they are commonly referred to, also are of little concern as they cannot reattach themselves to a new head of hair. Furthermore it should be noted that the majority of abandoned nits are damaged and never reach the stage of hatching, thus reducing the chances of exposure through this means. Even if they do manage to hatch, they require blood almost immediately or will starve to death.

An adult louse rarely leaves the security of a warm, generous host unless it has already identified a newer and more desirable environment to move onto. Since head lice feed every three to four hours they are unlikely to willingly leave their food supply.

It's also worth noting that lice prefer round shafts of hair because it's easier to wrap their claw-like feet around it. The hair of African-Americans is generally oval, a shape less maneuverable and thus less desirable to the louse. Lice also find curly hair less appealing. It's important to remember that although the shape of certain hair shafts reduces the risk of getting head lice, it does not make the person immune. With an increased number of interracial children, hair textures are changing, resulting in more cases of head lice among select racial groups than previously experienced.

Lice are more commonly found on girls than boys, presumably because their hair mass and longer length offer a more secure and attractive breeding ground. Additionally girls tend to be more physically affectionate than boys, resulting in more head-to-head contact. Longer hair, often found on girls, becomes a bridge of opportunity offering a mode of transportation from one head to another. The risk is increased if the child's hair is loose. The smaller volume of hair on most boys allows for more sun exposure, causing the skin to have a tougher texture and thus be a less inviting feeding ground for lice. Since head lice are lazy, they tend to look for a head that requires less work to obtain their needed food supply. I can't emphasize enough that while these reasons allow for more cases of head lice to be found on one gender and among certain races than others, it's no guarantee individuals in the less likely groups will be immune from them.

Why me?

There is some truth to the fact that certain people just seem to attract lice. While nothing personal, it's just that head lice are always on the lookout for a favorable environment. If you happen to be one of those unfortunate people - look out! You'll probably face more than your share of head lice infestations.

There are many factors that draw head lice to one individual over another. Blood type, particularly where the Rh factor is concerned, is among them. Head lice are amazingly intelligent. They have a sharp sense of smell and excellent eyesight. Head lice know what they need and will rarely move outside that environment. Only when faced with sure death do they cross over to an undesirable environment. Research has shown that lice avoid incompatible blood types unless they have reached the point of starvation. Even then, to feast on a new blood type can cause their intestinal tract to explode. While this sure means of death may slow down an infestation, it doesn't necessarily prevent one. Once a female louse crosses over, she will often lay her first batch of eggs prior to feeding. When the newly hatched nymphs feed on the new blood type, change in compatibility can occur.

Sometimes a louse will be fortunate enough to find a host that helps them travel between two more desirable environments. In this case the host serves as a bridge resulting in instances where there is an absence of live bugs and only a few eggs. The best way to explain it would be to picture a young child who has lice. Dad picks her up and she hugs him. In the process a bug crosses onto dad. He now puts that child down and before long picks up a second child. After laying a few eggs, the bug, not desiring Dad's head, moves off to the second child. In this case dad served as a bridge from one head to another.

Are children the only ones who get head lice?

Absolutely not! While it's more commonly spread among children, parents and other adults are not immune. If your child has head lice, you are at risk, as is any individual who has close contact with an infested child, including teachers, relatives and baby-sitters. Any time you curl up with the child, sit next to or lean over them, you are offering an opportunity for head lice to change environments. Keep in mind they are always looking for a new food supply. Likewise, as one host head becomes overcrowded, a louse will seek a new home.

When your hair has contact with another individual's hair (and it will), if that person has lice and you have a compatible environment, you are at risk of exposing yourself to an uninvited houseguest. Don't use this as a reason to not get close to the ones you love. Instead, to keep it safe, exercise common-sense precautions, such as tying your hair back.

Aren't lice a sign of being dirty?

This couldn't be farther from the truth! Head lice actually prefer clean hair - the cleaner the better. Since lice glue their eggs to the hair shaft, clean (non-oily) hair allows for easier attachment. It's far easier for lice to move around on clean hair, much like it is for you to walk on a clean floor versus a greasy one. It's worth noting that many home remedies to remove lice and nits are oil-based and transform the head into an undesirable environment. The belief that having lice means you're dirty is a myth that has gone on far too long.

Lice are equal opportunity parasites. They don't care about the size of your wallet, whether your house is clean or dirty or what your personal hygiene is. A louse's only concern is for its own survival. To accomplish this, the louse needs to feed and is always seeking the most convenient means of doing so.

It's worth adding that the only small truth to the "dirty environment" theory is that a dirty environment tends to be an undisturbed one. Head lice don't like to be disturbed. By combing, brushing, braiding and washing we are disturbing them; making our head less appealing. While a dirty head of hair is less desirable, one that is constantly disturbed is even worse to our unwanted friends. An example I frequently share with children in our office is: "If you are standing next to someone who is always pushing and punching you, you either want to punch that person back or you move away from them."

Will it help if I wash my child's hair daily?

This is nice in theory but unfortunately not true. Since nits are glued to the hair, all the brushing and washing on earth won't help. The eggs are coated with a fixative substance which literally cements them to the hair shaft, making nit removal a tedious and tiresome task. While you might "luck out" and wash a louse or two down the drain, don't count on it. Remember, these are blood-sucking parasites with crab-like claws, and they will hang on for dear life.

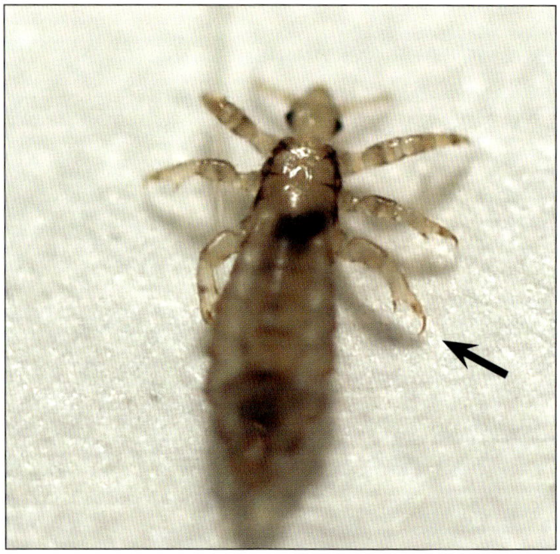

At the end of each leg are crab-like claws. Their claws allow them to tightly grasp on a strand of hair yet make it difficult for them to move on hard surfaces.

The fact is that lice are amazing critters. They have the ability to shut down their nervous systems and can remain submersed and unharmed for up to two hours, even in products intended to kill them. During laboratory testing, head lice have been found to play dead, only to move again when submersed for less than two hours.

Washing your child's hair is never a bad idea but understand that your reward is only going to be a clean head of hair. One more positive reason for taking such care is that you are disturbing their environment. The more you wash, brush or mess with the hair, the less desirable your head becomes to a visiting louse. Like us, they don't want to be in an environment where they can't rest or eat in peace, so we say: Comb, Wash, Brush, Braid--BE A PEST!

What about putting lots of gel on my child's hair?

I hear this question a lot and something I strongly discourage. Gel does nothing to prevent head lice. Used excessively gel will result in hair that looks bad and attracts every foreign particle that crosses its path. Many a misdiagnosis of lice has come about as a result of foreign matter in the hair that looked like lice but wasn't. It's far simpler to take a few extra minutes to brush the hair and pull it back, thus closing the bridge that invites a louse over.

How do I know for sure that my child has head lice?

There are many ways to know if your child has contracted a case of head lice. The most obvious way is the usual itchy scalp commonly (but not always) found in head lice cases. As the bug feeds, it secretes saliva, which keeps the blood from clotting, making its feeding process easier. As the saliva builds up, the itching "symptom" will most likely appear in ten to 14 days. The itching is an allergic reaction and, like most other allergies, not everyone reacts. As many as 50% of the individuals with head lice never itch. That said, just mention head lice and everyone itches! The only way to confirm your suspicions is with a thorough examination of your child's hair.

We need to also remember that head lice can lay eggs twice a day. Since they generally travel in harems, you'll end up with six, eight or even more head lice, with each female laying eight to ten nits a day! Just imagine how severe a case can become by the time you notice the itching. The best way to stay on top of this ever-increasing problem is by doing routine **head checks**. **Head checks** allow you to control the problem before it controls you. Making head lice exams part of your regular grooming routine allows you to identify the problem at its onset and prevent head lice from taking over your family, your home and your life.

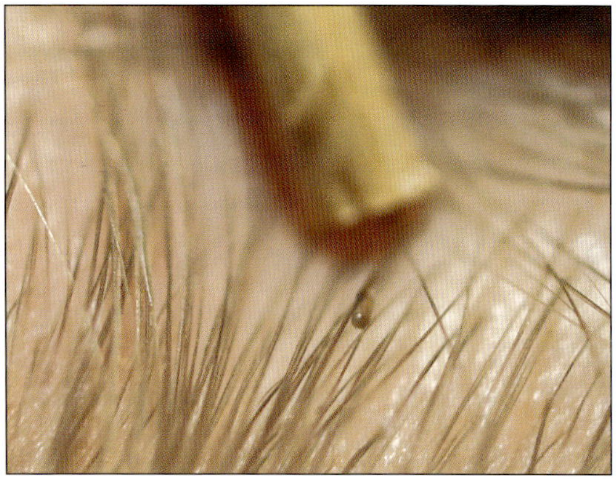

A nit "louse egg" is attached to the hair shaft with a fixative glue. Its cement-like substance will not dissolve and prevents nits from falling off the hair.

What if I find head lice?

If you find lice on your child's head, take care of the problem right away. Each day wasted is an increased opportunity for the lice to reproduce, worsening the infestation, and likely spreading it to others. Bear in mind that the fact that it spreads so easily is why you're dealing with this problem in the first place. Spreading not only occurs within the family but also among classmates, playmates and even out to strangers! A study conducted by Dr. Shirley Gordon and the Palm Beach County Head Lice Task Force in conjunction with Florida Atlantic University's School of Nursing defined "Persistent Head Lice" as three incidents of live lice found over a six-week period. Their research revealed that in the vast majority of cases another family member or close contact also had head lice. Obviously, this resulted in unknowingly handing it back and forth, similar to what happens with a bad cold.

How you treat the problem is entirely up to you. There are a lot of products on the market, but many are pesticides. If you feel you must use them, do so sparingly, and carefully follow all directions.

Whether you choose a pesticidal shampoo product or go with one of the newer non-toxic products, it is important to understand that 100% removal cannot occur without hours of painstakingly picking out all the nits. Sit down and make your child, as well as yourself, as comfortable as possible. You're going to be there for a while! Don't skimp on the process. There are no shortcuts. Make the time needed, and do it right. Remember, nits left behind are a chance for re-infestation. During your examination keep a watchful eye on the scalp as well, looking closely for nymphs. If you see what looks like a freckle or a speck of dirt, tap it. If it takes off running, it's a bug. Nymphs are often missed and are a large reason why lice infestations continue to exist. Left behind, they continue to grow, enabling a new generation of head lice to start the cycle all over again.

Thankfully, researchers have developd many new products to ease your burden. These include newer, more effective combs replacing the old plastic throw-away ones. Among this new generation of lice combs is the Terminator™. At an average cost of $12, this spiral tooth design is more effective in grabbing and removing nits, lessening the caregiver's burden and increasing the odds of a successful treatment. In a comb comparison study conducted by Lice Solutions Resource Network, Inc. in May 2006, the Terminator™ out-performed other leading combs as much as four to one. By using a good lice comb properly, you should expect to remove about 85% of the lice and nits.

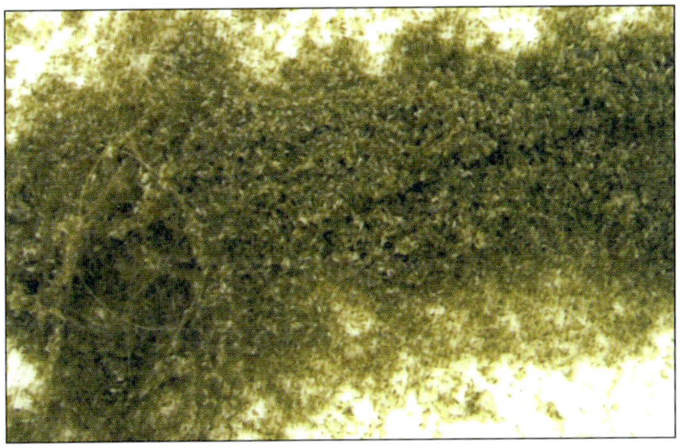

This photo shows hundreds of thousands of nits, combed out of one 12-year-old's hair after her mother claimed she had combed every day for two months. Had Mom had a better comb, she would have done a better job.

Another product that continues to draw attention is the Robi Comb™. Operating much like a bug zapper, the Robi Comb™ attacks the nervous system of any lice it comes into contact with. While the Robi Comb™ has proven helpful in eliminating live lice (particularly adults), it does little, if anything, to get rid of the nits. Since nits have yet to develop a nervous system, there is nothing for the comb to attack. It's an interesting concept but lacks efficiency. The unit retails for approximately $30, and if not used carefully or if applied to an extremely thick head of hair, it can run into mechanical problems. A similar product is the Magi Comb™. Also categorized as an electronic device, its design differs in that the teeth vibrate rather than the device sending an electronic current. With its close-set teeth, this device claims to help remove both lice and nits. It, too, sells for around $30, and while it may offer the user some relief, it still provides only partial elimination.

If the thought of all this is making you crazy, keep in mind that there are companies such as Lice Solutions that offer nit removal services. Since companies like ours provide this service on a regular basis, they can generally eliminate the problem faster and more efficiently than what most parents are able to accomplish at home. The fee charged by qualifed companies is often well worth it. Professionals are more likely to get the job done right the first time, in less time, and at a substantial savings compared to the parents' failed attempts to end their problem. If you are fortunate enough to have nit removal services in your area, don't hesitate to ask them questions about their qualifications and experience. After all, it is your child and your money.You have a right to know you're receiving the service you are paying for. Here are the common questions to ask:

How long have you been providing this service?
Where did you receive your training?
What method of nit removal do you use?
Is your **treatment process** safe?
What is your success rate?
Do you provide follow-up?
What guarantees, if any, do you offer?
What about other family members? Do you check them as well, and if so, is there an additional charge?

Be wary of any service that claims to have a 100% success rate, and remember - a truly efficient service will also examine the heads of all members of the family for the possibility of other cases within your household. By checking (and, if necessary, treating) all family members, you will have eliminated all possible sources within your household. Finally, if you're fortunate enough to have multiple resources in your community, make sure the one you choose is providing the most accurate, up-to-date lice information. If not, reconsider whether they are the right service to help you eliminate your head lice problem.

One last point, and probably the most important of all, is to be sure to notify everyone who has come into contact with anyone in your household who had an active case of head lice. Total eradication is not possible until all cases surrounding your family have been treated. There is nothing worse than working hard to eliminate a problem, only to have it handed back again.

How bad is the problem?

Head lice are among the most common reasons for absenteeism in schools across the country. While "No Nit Policies" come with good intentions (and are absolutely necessary), they have created an entirely new set of problems. Children with lice often miss school, causing their studies to suffer. Parents not only spend countless dollars on products (many of which don't work) but also often suffer the loss of income, due to missed work as well. Schools lose revenue, as most schools (particularly in public school settings) are funded on a per-head/per-day basis. This situation also causes damage to relationships between parents and administrators when schools diligently enforce their "No Nit Policy," adding hardship to the lives of the families battling head lice.

Further complicating matters is the fact that many school districts are moving entirely away from "No Nit Policies." Some are choosing instead to enforce a "Live Bug Only" policy, while others are choosing **no policy at all.** These are dangerous choices at best since ignoring a problem won't make it go away. Even the "Live Bug Only" policy now recommended by the American Academy of Pediatrics leaves a lot of parents scratching their heads for better answers. "Live Bug" means exactly that. Unless they find live bugs roaming through your child's hair, nits or not, they will be allowed to remain in school. This is a dangerous policy, since head lice are like chameleons and can blend with their environment, making it almost impossible for an untrained and inexperienced eye to see them. Many a child has entered our office with the nurse's assurance that he or she has nits but no bugs. The problem is that once we take the lice comb to the child's hair, we often comb out not one or two bugs, but rather 20 or more! It's a dangerous position and one that guarantees that head lice will continue to spread for years to come.

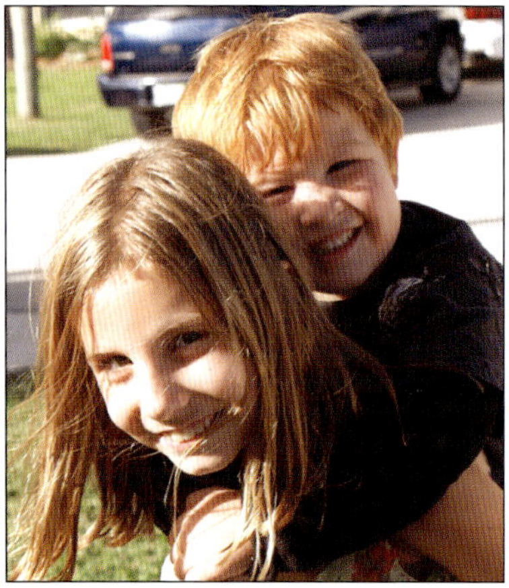

It's impossible to know exactly how many cases of head lice occur each year, but statistics from product sales suggest that the U.S. sees over 12 million cases of head lice annually. Head lice infestations in the U.S., are growing at epidemic proportions, its prevalence second only to the common cold.

When you consider the number of cases that go unreported, undetected, untreated, or are treated with home remedies, the number could be much higher. It is estimated that parents spend $150 million annually trying to eliminate this pesky parasite. The cost is far greater when you factor in lost wages that often occur as a result of parents being forced to miss work while tending to their child's head lice problem.

How bad is the problem? Bad enough to wreak havoc around the world! Bad enough to pit parents against school administrators. Bad enough for children to accept the blame and shame for a problem over which they have little control.

Why has this become such a problem?

In the past, if our child had head lice we treated them and sent them on their way, comfortable in the fact that **once treated,** both lice and nits were dead. However, newer research, brought about largely at the request of the National Pediculosis Association (NPA), a non-profit agency dedicated to protecting children from harmful lice **treatments**, has proven that methods utilized in the past are no longer effective.

Head lice are insects and, like other insects, can build up resistance over time to the products once effective in killing them. Another important reason head lice are harder to treat these days is that the problem perpetuates due to failure to follow through with precautionary measures. When you have treated your child's head you MUST incorporate additional safety measures to ensure you have eliminated all possible sources of re-exposure.

While the environment does not play as important a role as once thought, and mega cleaning is not necessary, you must still exercise common-sense cleaning. The best advice is to think of your life in a 24-hour window. Consider what items you had contact with in that time period, and keep your focus on those items only. You've been in bed, so you change your sheets. Either wash and dry them in hot temperatures or simply set them aside and replace with clean sheets. If the child sleeps with a stuffed animal or blanket, throw it in the dryer for 30 minutes. Run a light vacuum on the floors, over the sofa and on the child's favorite chair. If you do not have a vacuum with attachments, use a lint remover brush to collect loose hairs and possible bugs, or simply throw an old sheet over the area. Hairbrushes, combs, and recently used hair ties should be placed in boiling water for 15 minutes or soaked in ammonia, alcohol or dish detergent, as long as the items are submersed for at least two hours prior to re-use within that 24 hour window.

Keep in mind that while these steps are important, you shouldn't become consumed with the cleaning process. Remember, lice DO NOT live in your home. The problem is on your head and the heads of those around you. The risk that parents are not removing all of the lice and nits from the child's hair is far greater than the risk of exposure from the environment. It's not uncommon for a parent to shampoo and comb a child's hair, only to find the child re-infested a week later. This is largely due to the fact that remaining nits were not killed. If nits are left on the hair to hatch, the cycle starts over again.

Equally important is the need to recognize and remove all nymphs. Often as tiny as the tip of a sharp pencil, nymphs grow to start families of their own. Sadly, however, little is said about the nymphs, and while many parents may diligently search out nits, they fail to recognize the importance of removing the nymphs. Finally, don't forget that the greatest source of re-infestation is people with whom the infested person has had contact. We like to say, "It's the gift that keeps on giving." Certainly **not** a gift any of us hope for, it is nonetheless a huge factor in why families struggle to get past head lice. Keep in mind it's not just about where you got head lice but also to whom you gave it as well.

While resistance issues are a large factor in the increased number of head lice infestations, they are far from being totally responsible. As the pharmaceutical companies are quick to point out, the directions on the package are there for a reason. Unless you are willing to read and follow them in their entirety, you can't expect the products to end the problem.

Keep in mind that head lice need blood to survive, so the best use of your time is checking and combing your child's head and communicating with those around you. Doing so is far more important than stripping your sheets, vacuuming three times a day and bagging every toy your child owns. Nit removal is a tedious enough job without overburdening yourself with unnecessary cleaning tasks. It's not necessary to drive yourself into a state of hysteria or have a nervous breakdown in an attempt to regain a normal lifestyle.

One final note, **but most important of all**, is to keep in mind how this affects your child. We don't want children to feel that it's their fault or to be ashamed because they have head lice. It happens! We must stress that to the children. We must be willing to deal with it, get over it and go on with our lives.

Is there any danger?

For the most part, head lice are simply an irritating problem. While their saliva can produce an allergic reaction in certain individuals, these reactions are generally mild compared to the potential risk involved with many lice shampoo products.

Products containing lindane have caused the greatest concerns. In August of 2006 the United States joined more than 50 other countries in banning the use of lindane. Exposure to the neurotoxic product has been linked to seizures, developmental disabilities, hormone disruption and worse yet—cancer. Thanks to the Environmental Protection Agency (EPA), one can no longer treat animals or the environment with lindane, as it is considered too dangerous. The only use still allowed is as an ingredient in shampoos and lotions for the **treatment** of head lice and scabies. Since the Food and Drug Administration (FDA) and not the EPA oversees these products, they continue to be made available. Thankfully many states, including California, New York and Michigan, have taken this decision out of the FDA's hands and banned its use within their states.

Adding to the danger of lindane is the fact that many people fail to follow the directions properly, leaving the shampoo on longer than recommended or re-treating too quickly. Improper use is one of the biggest causes of treatment failure and among the greatest dangers to your child. Another danger, and one clearly explained on many shampoo labels, is treating a child under the age of two or the use of such products by pregnant women. In 2005 French researchers discovered that pregnant women who used insecticides almost doubled the risk of their child developing acute leukemia.

Another risk, and one that should be obvious but is sometimes ignored, is using treatment products on individuals with scalp irritations. Unfortunately, parents' desperate and overzealous attempts to eliminate their child's head lice infestation often puts their child at risk of far greater harm.

Finally, let's not forget that many of the lice remedies contain other pesticides. While the FDA has approved some products as safe to use on children, many parents prefer not to expose their children to pesticides if there is another alternative. It's YOUR child's head; is this really how you want to deal with the problem? For these reasons Lice Solutions uses only non-toxic lice shampoos and relies on combing procedures, not chemicals, to eliminate head lice on the individual's we treat. Work to get rid of the pesky critters, but always do so in a safe and effective manner.

What is being done about it?

The NPA was formed in 1982. Since then the association has made great strides in increasing awareness through research and education. The group fought to limit the use of potentially harmful products containing dangerous chemicals such as lindane and was also instrumental in formulating the "No Nit Policy" utilized in many schools. This non-profit agency, dedicated to protecting children from harmful lice **treatments**, was also instrumental in recognizing the importance of combing. As a result of their research, they have helped revolutionize the way we treat head lice, through better and more effective combs.

Extensive research has also been conducted in an effort to find safer and more effective means for dealing with this so called new breed of "super louse." Joining the efforts in the quest for better answers are top lice researchers like John Clark, Ph.D., a toxicologist with the Department of Veterinary Animal Sciences at the University of Massachusetts. Dr. Clark has conducted extensive research on resistance issues and has developed the first system for breeding head lice off of the head, an important tool in his ongoing efforts to better understand head lice.

Likewise, Ian Burgess, an entomologist and Chief Investigator, Medical Entomology Centre, Insect R&D Limited in Cambridge, England, has seen more than his share of product failures. In one study on permethrin products, he found only a 78% success rate after two treatments. A study two years later along the same lines showed a mere 55% success rate after two treatments. Another researcher leading the industry is Dale Clayton, Ph.D., Professor of Biology at the University of Utah and Founder & Chief Scientific Officer, Larada Sciences, Inc., has gone a step further by developing a hot air device he hopes will help families as he seeks better ways to deal with this newer breed of resistant head lice. Much has been said about this new "super louse," a catch-all phrase that refers not to a new breed of lice, but rather a stronger, more resistant form of head lice.

Another important step towards dealing with this problem is the banding together of concerned parents to form organizations dedicated to helping fight this pesky parasite. While great strides have been made in the fight against head lice, it's still not enough. Only by continuing to band together, by speaking up for more proactive measures in your schools and your community, can you help prevent head lice from escalating in your area.

How can I help?

There are many ways to help, and organizations such as Lice Solutions are always looking for those willing to lend a hand.

For starters, check in your local area to determine if there are any organizations working towards the education and elimination of head lice. If so, make yourself available to assist in any way possible. If not, consider starting a small group in your area. Look for individuals who are equally frustrated, and band together to promote proactive and preventive measures. It's not an easy fight but is a battle worth fighting.

If you are unable to locate a facility in your area, contact our non-profit organization, Lice Solutions Resource Network, Inc. at (561) 842-9969 and ask if we are aware of any organizations close to you or how you might be able to help bring services to your area. Our goal as a non-profit organization is to one day have Lice Solutions' facilities in major cities across the U.S. It's individuals like you who will help make that possible. Only by ensuring that ***all*** children receive the help they need can we possibly hope to keep ***our*** children safe from head lice infestations.

So, how can you make a difference in your school? First, confirm that your school is operating under a "No Nit Policy." If not, let them know that you believe that only through proactive policies can you hope to eliminate head lice in your school. Find other parents who agree with you, and meet with your school nurse, principal or the school board if necessary to bring about change. Identify what your school's policy is regarding notification of parents when head lice have been identified in your child's classroom. If no notification exists, ask why and what you can do to help develop more proactive measures.

In Palm Beach County, Florida the Head Lice Task Force Team believes that notification works against the problem. This group has found a direct correlation between the notification of head lice infestations and increased product sales of lice-related items. It is the team's belief that many parents prophylactically treat at times of outbreaks in hopes of preventing possible infestation. Whether increased sales are a result of prophylactic **treatments** or actual cases of head lice is hard to say. One good thing that has come out of this panel's efforts is a recommendation that could definitely reduce the number of cases seen each year. It is the panel's belief that if every parent of a school-aged child had a good lice comb and used it (for two to five minutes on wet hair) once or twice a week, lice would not be a problem, because the problem would be identified at first onset before escalating and spreading to others. Unfortunately school administrators in Palm Beach County have yet to implement this suggestion and therefore failed to share this valuable information with their parents.

Preventive combing is a great recommendation. Now we just need more schools incorporating it and more parents acting on it. It's a wonderful solution and one I always suggest to the families that visit our facility. If I had my way, a good lice comb would be on the school supply list of every school in the country.

Only through improved "No Nit Policies," as well as parents and school administrators working together, can we hope to bring about a positive end to this ever-increasing problem. Remember, you're in a potentially "no-win" situation. If you rid your child of head lice only to return the child to an environment that is not being checked, you're pretty much guaranteed to be dealing with it again and again. While you may not be able to change the school's stand on head lice policies, you can develop proactive measures within your household.

Become an advocate for head lice and encourage regular screenings not only in your child's classroom but in the entire school as well. It is in the best interests of the student body to require at least three screenings per year. Whether your school checks heads once a year or five times a year, the school should also develop protocols to ensure that all of the children's heads were in fact checked. Because some children may be absent on that particular day, ask the administration to set a mandate that each absent child must go through the school nurse's office for a **head check** prior to entering their classroom. Be sure that the administration bring the teachers on board to assist with enforcement of this policy. While this may seem like overkill, parents have admitted to us that they intentionally kept their children home on days the school had scheduled **head checks**. One such example involved a nurse's daughter. The nurse shared that for four years her family battled head lice, and while the school did head **checks** regularly, she taught her daughter to be an expert at avoiding them. This mom stated, "If I knew they were doing a **head check** that day, she'd stay home 'sick.' If it was a surprise **head check**, she'd ask to go to the bathroom to avoid being checked." Only when the case had escalated to the point that Mom could visibly see bugs crawling around her daughter's hair, did she decide it was time to get help. You can be fairly certain that those who protest the most or tend to avoid **head checks** are the same ones who have head lice and know it.

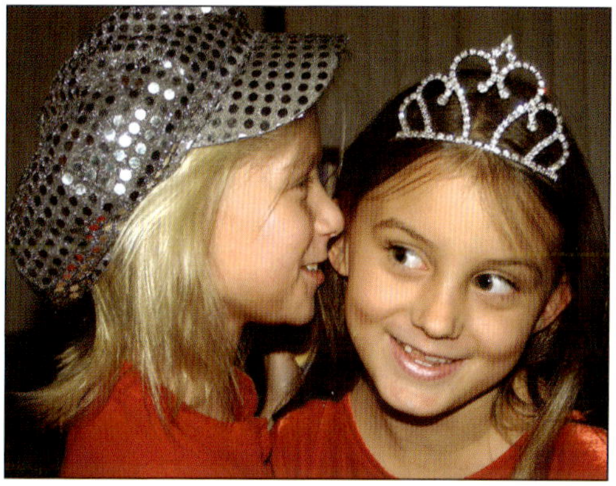

As you move forward, ask the school to incorporate a policy on how to handle cases found in the future. Should head lice be found on one child, all close contacts must be checked as well. This includes classmates, siblings, relatives, and close friends. Only by establishing more proactive measures can you hope to reduce the number of cases seen in your school each year.

So, what times of the year should schools' schedule school wide **head checks**? A good rule of thumb for regular screenings is at the beginning of each school year, after winter break, and prior to releasing students for summer vacation. In doing so, you'll reduce the overall number of infestations by stopping the spread of head lice, and you'll help reduce the odds of your child's school having an epidemic.

The first week of August is **Head Check** Awareness Week. This is the perfect time for parents to add **head checks** to their "To-Do List." Lice Solutions does its part by offering free **head checks** the entire week to <u>any child</u> entering our facility. By doing so we hope to help reduce the number of cases entering our schools each year.

It can't stop there, however. Parents must be notified if an outbreak exists in their child's class. They should work with the schools by checking their child's head daily for the three weeks following an outbreak. These checks need only take a few minutes a day and could save countless hours later on. Early detection is the key to minimizing transmission among students. For schools dealing with a head lice problem, we encourage them to check the heads of the infested child's siblings as well. It serves little purpose to rid one classroom of head lice if a brother or sister is sharing head lice in another. This can be done quickly and discreetly. If that child is clear, send him or her back to class; if not, start the entire process in that classroom. If not taken seriously it can quickly snowball into a major epidemic; dealt with properly, however, you can stop head lice in its tracks!

To further emphasize how severe a neglected problem can get, I'd like to share a story with you.

Several years ago, one of our local middle school nurses called about a seventh grader who was battling a head lice problem. The school was well aware of it, but since the child had already missed so much school, she was allowed to continue attending class. What the school wasn't aware of was the severity of the situation. Our technician, ill-prepared for how drastic the problem was, quickly had to call for reinforcements. The child's head was so infested that it took two technicians four hours each, and even then they couldn't get them all.

Because her head lice had been neglected for so long, it was difficult to work on her tender scalp. Not only was her hair matted to her scalp but she also suffered multiple open wounds that had blood and puss oozing from them. The technicians worked diligently, each taking a side of the child's head, gently attempting to remove as many of the lice and nits as possible. The advanced state of the infestation as well as the lack of care required them to wash the child's hair three times just to soften it enough to work with it. Hundreds of live lice literally ran from her hair, and there were few strands not filled with nits.

Finally the technicians had done all they could. To do more would require medical treatment. After a conference call with zoologist and renowned lice expert Terri Meinking, as well as a local pediatrician, a follow-up course of action was determined that included antibiotics to heal the sores and kill off the remaining lice. It also became a child-neglect issue, since the situation should never have reached that proportion. Mom, knowing the child had head lice, felt that at 12 years of age she should have been old enough to tend to her own head.

It also became a serious school problem. Upon notification to her school nurse, they did a head by head check of the entire seventh grade and sent 86 children home in one day. We dropped out of the loop before hearing exactly how many more children they found as they searched the remaining grades. On a positive note, it was amazing how much better her hair looked when our technicians completed their job, an appearance change that had a positive impact on her self esteem. While I know this description has probably made your stomach turn, it's important to understand how quickly a neglected case of head lice can become a severe problem.

Should you determine that your child has head lice, get busy and treat it. Keep the child away from playmates until you do so, and notify anyone who has had recent contact with your child. Battling head lice is an inconvenience for everyone involved, especially for the individual afflicted with the problem, and it only gets worse if ignored. If you are among the unfortunate millions to receive a home visit from this uninvited guest, speak up. Be a friend and tell your friends to have their hair checked. Notify the school, clubs and organizations, church, daycare and anyone else your child has had contact with. Keep in mind that symptoms are generally not noticeable until seven to ten days after infestation. Don't allow the problem to escalate or spread before you begin proactive measures.

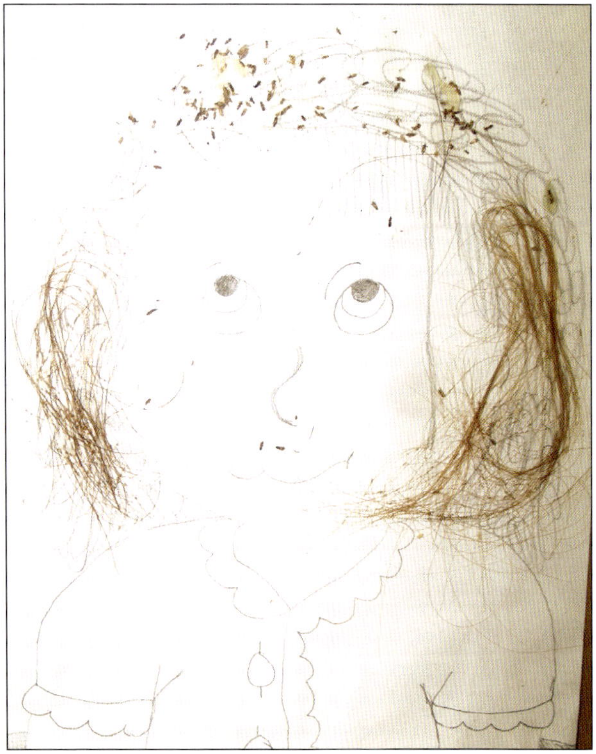

This drawing, displayed in our office, depicts how severe an infestation can become. The drawing contains actual bugs and nits removed from the head of the twelve year old mentioned in my story.

Do you really want your child's hair to look like this?

Understand that telling others is a necessary process to ensure that your child does not get it back again. Your child came in contact with head lice somewhere and will surely spread it to others before you realize your child has it. Treating your child and then returning them to a possible lice-infested environment is asking for trouble. Communicate with everyone involved and help put an end to the cycle.

Finally if you are unfortunate enough to become a member of the double-whammy club, remember this important fact, "If you must re-treat, change prducts." In doing so, you will reduce the chances of dealing with a resistance problem. Carefully follow the directions on the package, leaving the product on only for the required time and allowing adequate time between **treatments**. Also don't forget to check other family members, as well as close friends. Remember, just like a bad cold it will spread just as quickly.

The most important factor that can't be stressed enough is that having head lice should be no more embarrassing than having chicken pox. As parents, we're sorry for those to whom we unknowingly spread it, but it happens. We need to stop the blame game. That means don't look to blame, and don't stress over being blamed. *Head lice happens*! The only fault you can claim is if you fail to act when you become aware of the situation. We always tell our families, "It's not just about where you got head lice but who you gave it to as well. " Get over the blame game, accept that it happens, and deal with the problem.

In an effort to better document cases and localities, we ask your help in reporting these cases to our facility. We work with several universities, providing them with data for their ongoing research. To contact Lice Solutions, e-mail us at info@licesolutions.org, or call us at (561) 842-9969.

Are you uncertain as to whether you have head lice or not? Send us your samples. We will examine them under a microscope and let you know what we find. Although a suggested donation of $10 is encouraged, there is no required fee for this service.

Many an unnecessary **treatment** could have been avoided if the time had been taken to confirm head lice prior to treating. When sending samples, either place them in a Ziploc bag, or afix them with Scotch tape onto a sheet of white paper. Be sure to include your name, telephone number, and location, along with the name, sex, and age of the individual from whom the samples were removed. Mail the envelope to Lice Solutions, 6758 North Military Trail, Suite #110, West Palm Beach, Florida 33407. We generally call back the same day we receive the sample.

Lastly, remember to add Lice Solutions Resource Network, Inc. to your list of favorite charities. As we tell clients daily, we are not federally funded--we're publicly funded. We cannot exist without your donations. Please also remember us when considering your annual charitable contributions. Take advantage of any matching programs that your company might offer. If you belong to any organizations that provide fundraising activities to benefit local and national charities, please ask them to add us to their list as well. We ask that you help us, so that we may continue to help you.

Head lice are never pleasant, but there is help you can count on. "Head Lice Happens. Get over it and move on!" Now thanks to Lice Solutions, getting rid of head lice has never been easier.

2

WHAT TO EXPECT

Terminology can sometimes be confusing to the novice user. Therefore I want to help you understand the process involved and the sequential steps it entails.

You have reason to suspect that your child has head lice - *now what*?

1. **Head check** - examination of child's head and hair to determine if lice or nits are present.

2. **Treatment** - if lice or nits are found, product should be applied and a thorough **treatment** to remove all lice and nits administered. **Treatment** starts with an **initial comb-out** and ends with a **final re-check.**

3. **Initial comb-out** - actively combing through hair to remove as many lice and nits as possible prior to manual **nit picking.**

4. **Nit picking** - the manual removal of lice and nits, usually done in a **strand-by-strand** process throughout the hair.

5. **Final re-check** - done upon completion of **treatment** to ensure nothing was missed during the **treatment process.** This is most effective on dry hair.

6. **Final comb-out** - combing of the hair with additional product upon completion of **final re-check.** Especially critical if newly hatched nymphs exist, as they live directly on the scalp and will blend with their environment.

7. **Follow-up re-check** - the examination of the treated individual's hair in the days and weeks following **treatment**. Can be done any time after **treatment** but should be no more than seven days later. **Follow-up re-checks** should be continued for at least 14 days after **treatment** and stopped only after two clean **re-checks,** with no further lice or nits found. **Follow-up re-checks** are necessary to ensure all lice and nits have been removed and that no further contact with other active cases of head lice exist.

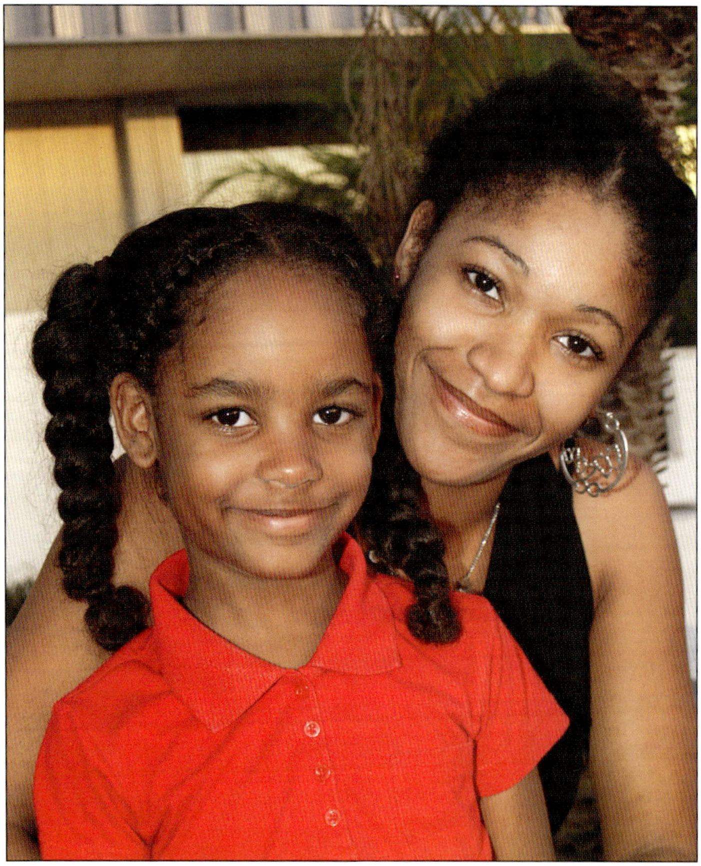

3

HEAD CHECK PROCEDURES

For short haired individuals, see procedures on page 39 adapted for that length of hair.

Tools Used: detangler comb, wooden stick, lice comb, non-toxic mint spritz, and hair tie. (Not all of these tools may be needed.) To purchase needed items, check your local pharmacy, beauty supply store or visit: www.licesloutions.org.

Purpose: In an attempt to avoid unnecessary **treatments,** we recommend checking heads prior to any **treatment process**. Every individual in the household should be checked to determine if they, too, have any **evidence** of head lice. ***Evidence** is considered to be nits and/or bugs*.

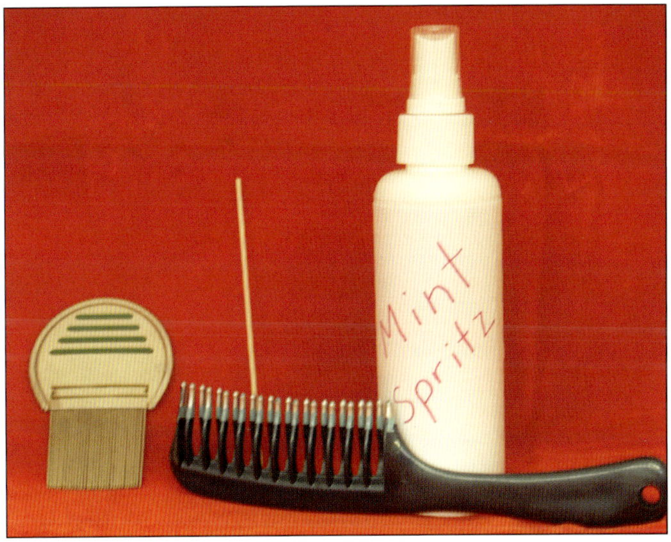

From left to right: Quality lice comb, detangler comb, wooden stick, and mint spritz

I have found the best combs to be all metal, allowing the teeth to be welded in for durability. The teeth should be closely positioned in a manner that prevents seeing through the comb. Spiral microgrooved tines offer an added bonus, and an anti-slip band or similar mechanism assures a firm grip during the treatment process.

When checking for nits or bugs, it is important to work with thin layers of hair. Primary areas of focus are nearest the scalp. **Head checks** start at the bottom of the neck area and move upward in thin layers until the top of the head has been reached. If the individual being examined has bangs, check that area separately and only upon completing the examination of the bulk of the head of hair. If **evidence** is found at any time during the **head check**, the parent or caregiver should stop immediately, as **treatment** is deemed necessary. Examination of the entire head is not necessary once the presence of head lice is identified.

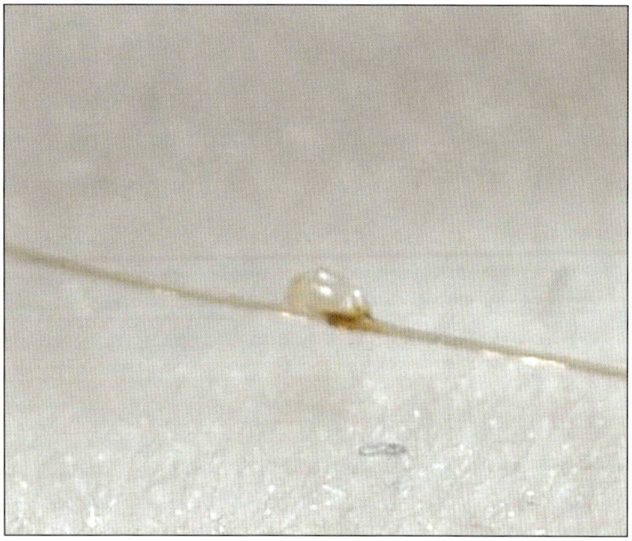

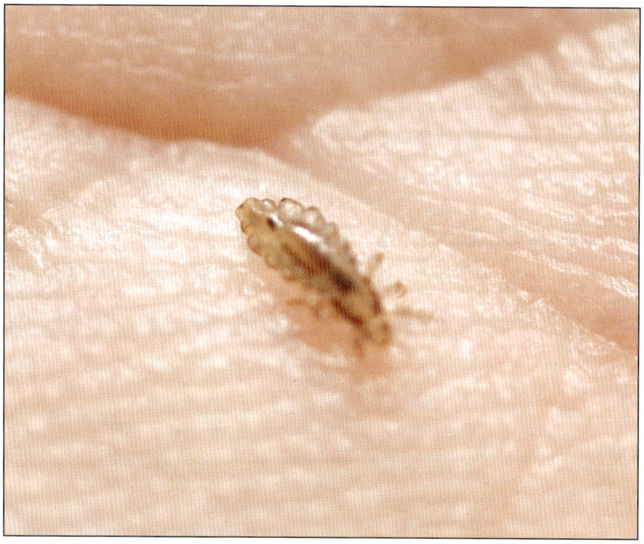

Evidence - On the left is a nit on the hair, while the right shows a live louse in the hand of our technician. Such **evidence** is removed and shown to the caregiver for verification of head lice.

A head check for longer hair consists of the following steps:

Comb the tangles out of the hair with a detangler comb. Remember that if **evidence** is found, the parent or caregiver should stop checking the head at that time.

At the Lice Solutions offices we require our technicians to remove a strand of hair with the nit attached, or remove a bug if found, and show any **evidence** to the individual being examined. Most people feel a sense of comfort knowing that the **treatment** is justified. I encourage you to do the same when checking for head lice at home. I recommend that you tape your sample to a white sheet of paper or place it in a Ziploc bag if there is any doubt that this is in fact lice related.

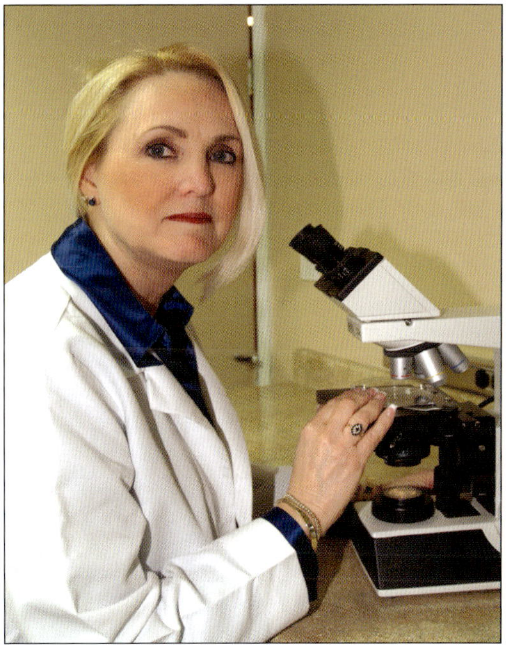

Katie Shepherd, Founder & CEO of *The Shepherd Institute for Lice Solutions*.

Our office encourages parents to mail samples to the West Palm Beach facility. Samples are generally viewed under a microscope the same day that they are received. Should you choose to send us samples, be sure to include the individual's first name, age, gender and contact information. After samples have been examined, one of our staff members will call you with the results. Although a suggested donation of $10 is encouraged, there is no required fee for this service.

"Not sure what you are looking at? Send us a sample and we'll let you know what it is!"

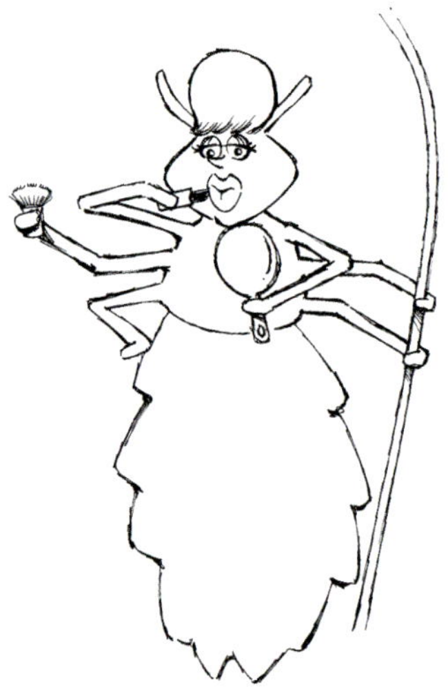

We feel strongly that proper identification must be made to help prevent unnecessary **treatments** and recommend that **treatment** be administered only if **evidence** is found. (An exception to this rule would be if this is considered a **follow-up re-check** and you found a few missed nits. In such cases follow the directions in the chapter on **follow-up re-check**s.) Good vision is a prerequisite for the diagnosis of head lice infestations, as nits and particularly nymphs can be very difficult to see. If a lice **treatment** facility is available in your area, you may want to consider contacting them for help.

Once you have combed the hair free of tangles, grasp the hair with one hand and position it high on the head much like an imaginary ponytail. The hair is held in this manner during the entire check or until **evidence** is found. Using your free hand, pull down thin layers of hair with your fingernail, wooden stick or similar tool (this is a personal preference), working your way towards the top of the head. You will be examining both the scalp and the hair during this process. Bugs will often appear as a speck of dirt on the scalp, or you might note a bug in movement. Nits, on the other hand, are attached to the strand of hair. They do not move easily along the hair shaft. You might also notice something glistening, particularly in bright lighting. Eggs (or nits as they are commonly called) tend to be reflective, similar to a mirror in sunlight.

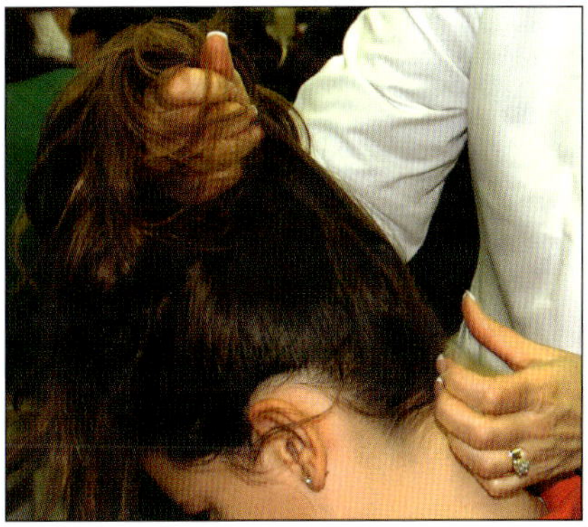

Holding the hair in an imaginary ponytail ensures a more thorough and accurate **head-check** process.

Begin by pulling thin layers of hair from the bottom of the neck area, around the ears and sideburns. Continue pulling thin layers, moving from one side of the head to the other and around the neck area. Moving back and forth allows you to work through any tangles. As you work your way through the hair, keep your eyes focused on both the hair and the scalp areas, watching for **evidence** of lice. For those with vision difficulties, magnifying headsets are available for a minimal cost to assist with this task. (Reminder: If any **evidence** is found at any time, STOP! **Treatment** is now warranted.)

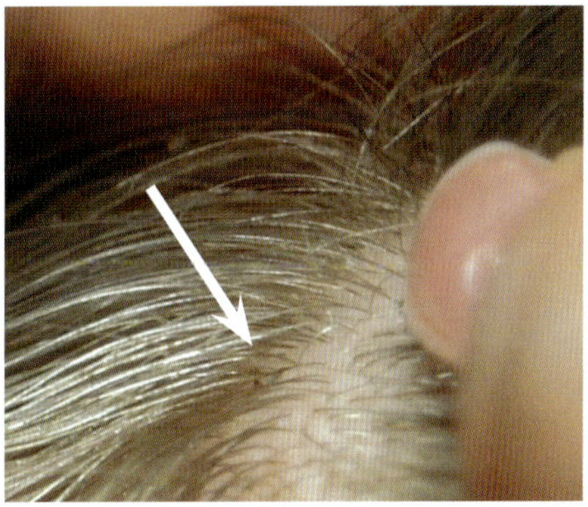

Nymphs look like a freckle or speck of dirt and live directly on the scalp.

Continue pulling thin layers from side to side, moving evenly upward around the head. You will be working your way

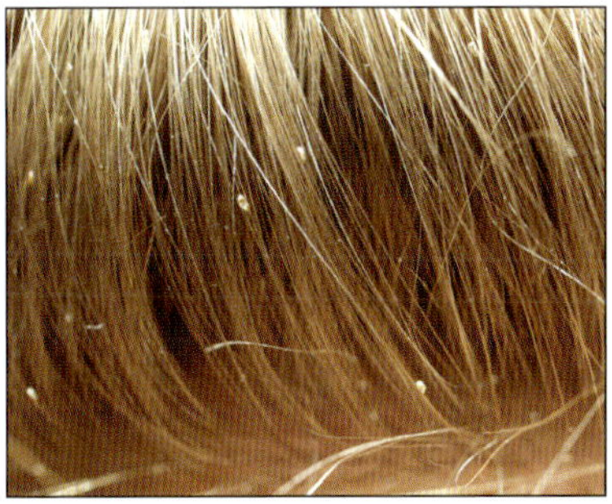

The task of spotting nits simplifies as the quantities of nits increase. You'll also note in this picture how they tend to glisten, aiding parents in their search.

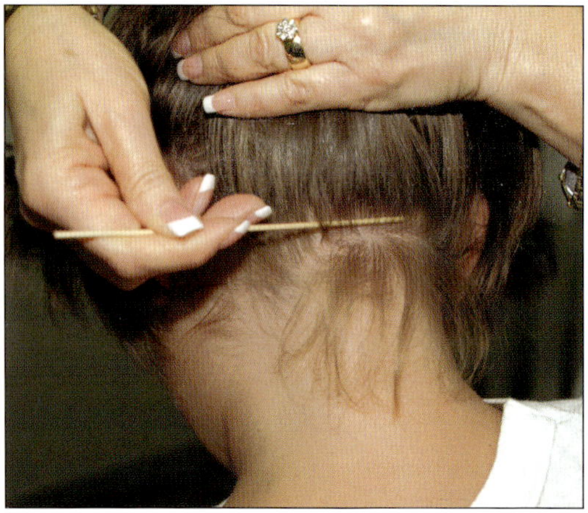

Start your **head-check** at the nape of the neck. Be careful to examine both the hair and the scalp.

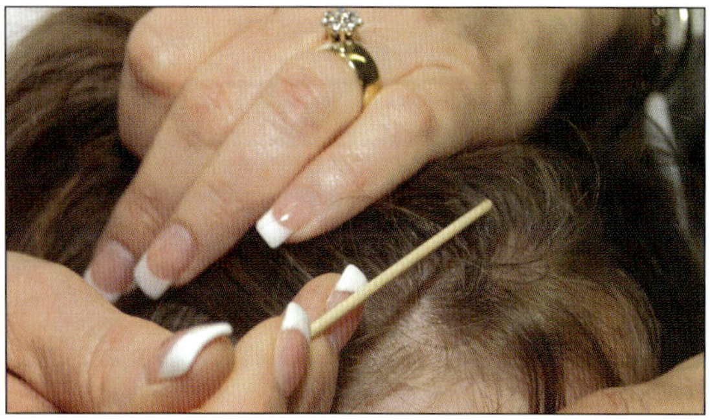

Bangs are a favorite place for lice to lay their eggs.

to the top of the head, pulling down thin layers of hair until there are no more layers to be checked. If the individual has bangs, it is now time to check them. Begin by holding the bangs up with one hand or simply pushing them back, holding them down in the process. Start checking bangs by pulling thin layers forward until there are no more layers left to examine.

Next, provide the individual you are checking with a paper towel to cover their eyes. Ask them to tilt their head back. With their head back, spray a non-toxic mint spritz lightly around the head. The spritz will assist in the combing process. Additionally, mint is an offensive odor to the bugs and will cause them to run, increasing the chances of finding them. Use the lice comb for two to three minutes and comb at a 90-degree angle. Starting at the scalp, comb hair in multiple directions using backward, downward and upward motions. Be certain to comb all the way through the hair to the ends of the hair shaft. If a bug exists, removing the comb prior to reaching the end of the hair could result in a bug being left behind. During this **comb-out**, be careful to check the comb often for **evidence**. Again, if **evidence** is found at any time, STOP! Inform the individual that **treatment** is needed.

If no **evidence** is found, comb the hair back with a detangler comb and put hair into a ponytail, braid or similar safe style. They are good to go for another week.

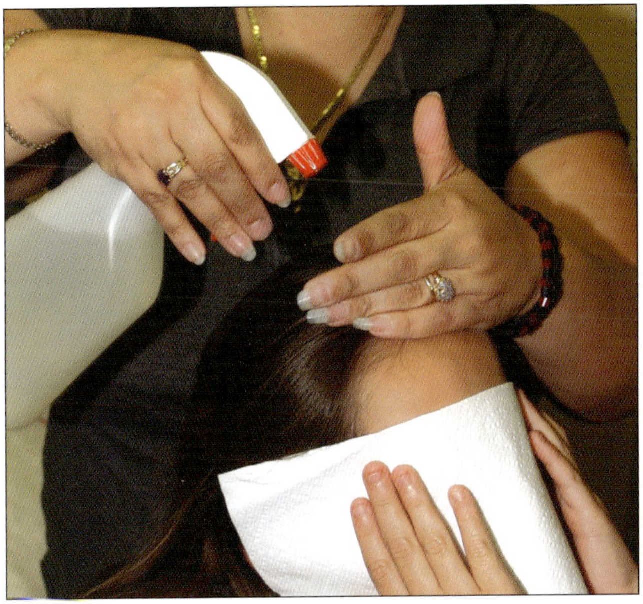

Be careful to keep the head back when applying any product and **always protect their eyes!**

Bottom left: Be sure to comb all the way to the end of hair to make certain all bugs are removed.

Bottom: Combing at a 90 degree angle assures a more successful **comb-out** process.

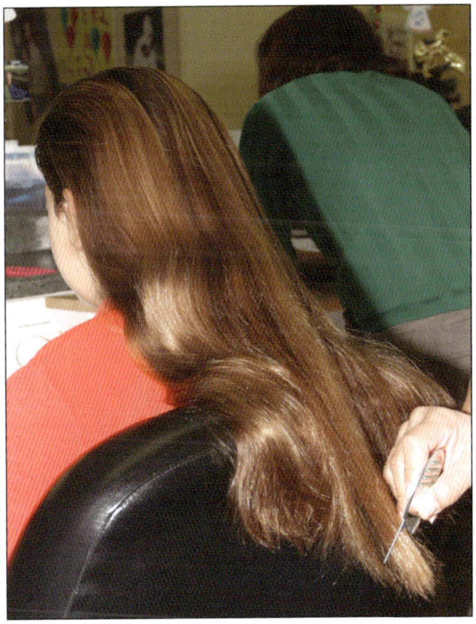

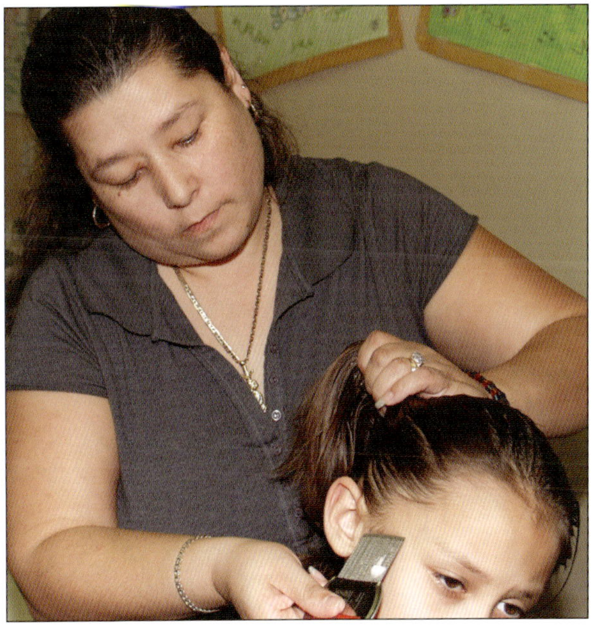

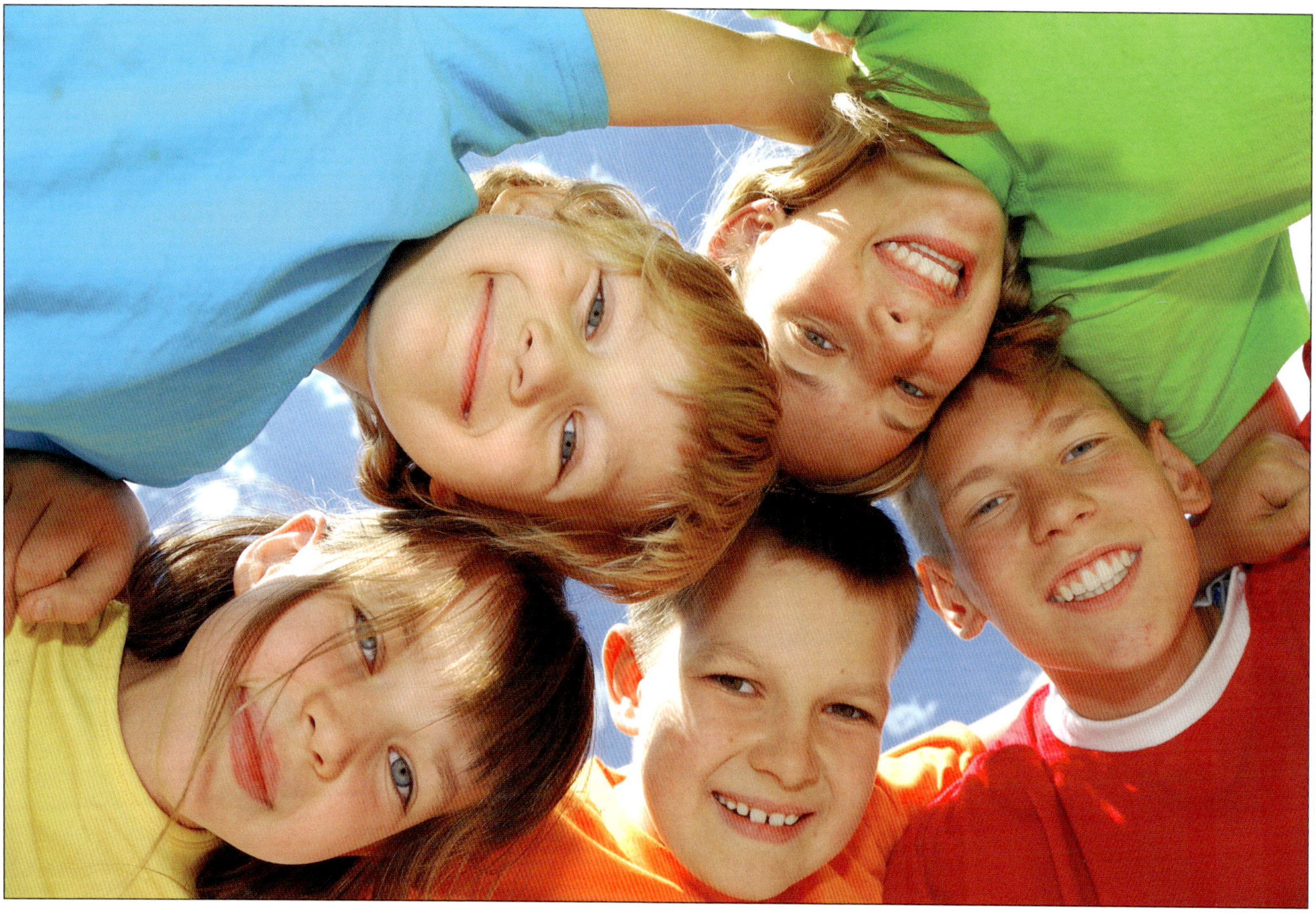

SHORT HAIR HEAD CHECKS – A UNIQUE APPROACH

The method on short-haired individuals is somewhat different than that for longer hair. Depending upon the individual's length of hair, the hair can be checked in either thin layers or small sections. Keep in mind that this technique is used when working with hair that is too short to grasp. On extremely short hair, as would be the case with the cropped hair of many boys, the **head check** will start at the top of the head. I strongly encourage you to always adhere to the recommended steps, as being systematic ensures that all the hair was examined. (Reminder: If any **evidence** is found at any time, STOP! Inform the individual you are checking that **treatment** is needed.)

A **head check** for shorter hair consists of the following steps:

Comb the tangles out of the hair with a detangler comb.

With your left hand (assuming you are right-handed) hold hair back at the forehead. As you hold the hair down, take your right hand and pull thin layers of hair forward. If the individual has longer hair (but still too short to grasp all at once) grasp one section at a time - similar to the bangs technique). Depending on the length, pull the hair forward in thin layers or small sections with your fingernail, a wooden stick, or similar tool (this is a personal preference). Continue to pull thin layers or small sections of hair while simultaneously moving towards the crown of the head. When the crown area is reached, this part is done.

Next, begin checking the sides of the head. Generally, we prefer to check the right side of the head first (by checking the same way each time, there is no doubt that you have checked every area) although it does not matter which side is done first, as long as both sides are checked thoroughly. The sides are checked from the sideburns, around the ears, moving upward in the same manner applied in the previous step.

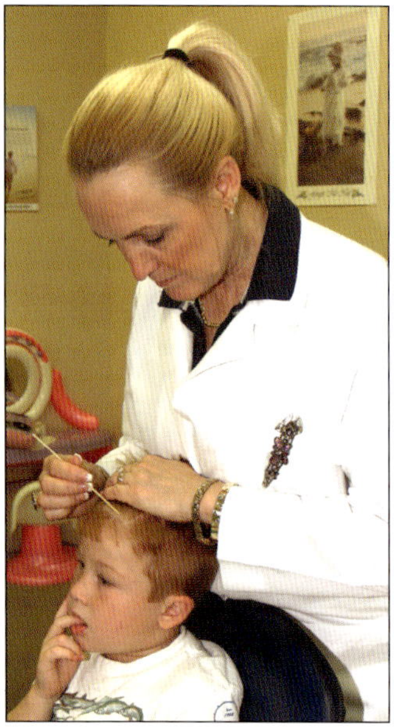

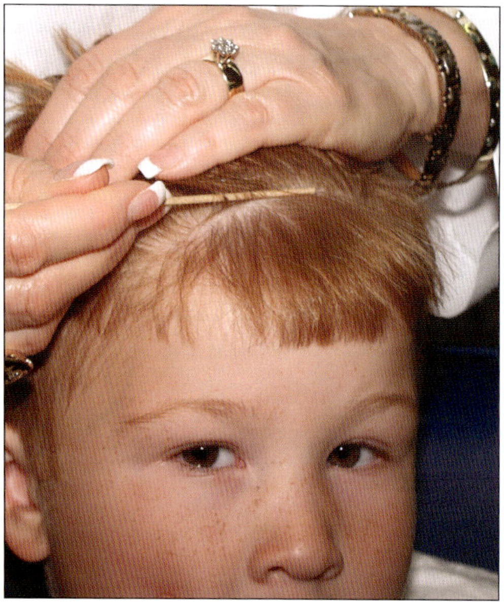

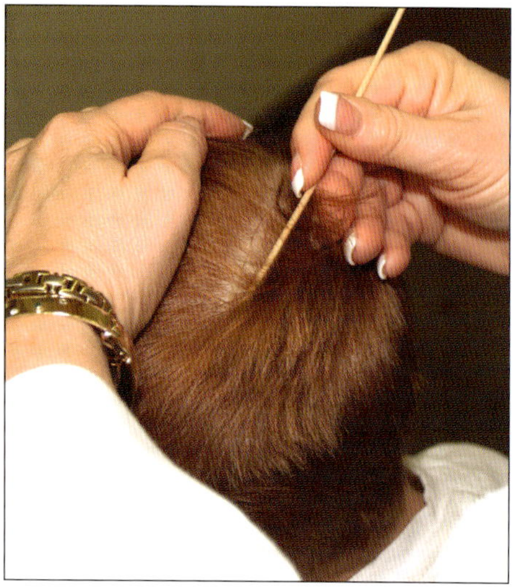

The method of checking short hair is unique... you start at the forehead and work towards the crown. Top left is checking short hair at the forehead. Middle is a close-up showing Ms. Shepherd using her left hand to hold the short hair back while going through the hair in paper thin layers. Right shows her checking the crown area.

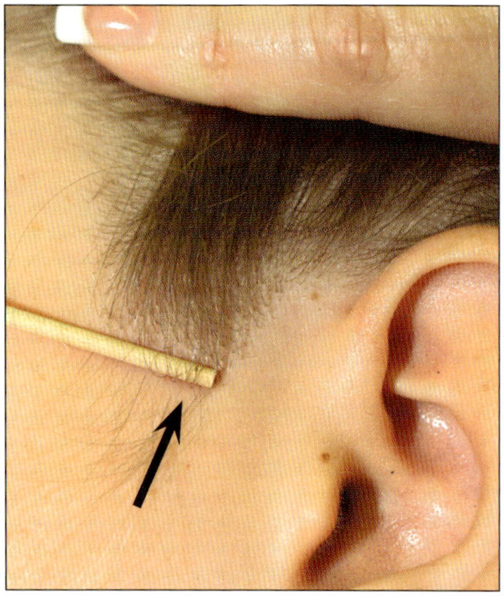

Check the sideburns carefully, as this is a favorite place for lice to hide their eggs.

Place one hand on the side of the head near the sideburn and gently pull down thin layers of hair. Again, if hair is more than 2" long, you may grasp the section and pull down hair as would be done with the imaginary ponytail technique. When the top of the head is reached, this part is done. Continue the same technique for the opposite side of head. Be extra cautious in your search, as this is a popular area for lice to lay their eggs.

Moving on to the back of the head, ask the person to tilt his/her head forward. Placing one of your hands at the back of their neck, push the hair upward. Repeat the process utilized in previous hair sections. Begin by pulling thin layers or small sections from one side of the head to the other and move up towards the top of the head. Once you reach the top of the head, this part is completed. Be careful to take extra time at the nape of the neck, as some individuals have deep indentations, making this a popular area for bugs to lay their eggs, and more difficult for you to search.

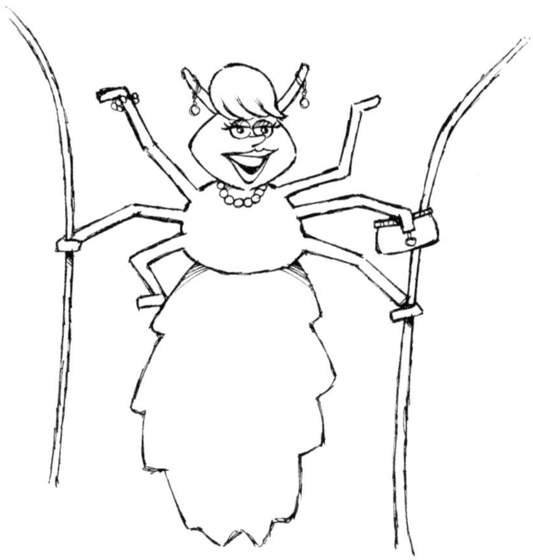

"Did you know that you have "Hot Spots" on your head? Hot spots are areas where lice like to lay their eggs. These are the crown area, around the ears, the nape of the neck and the bang area."

Finally, examine the back side behind the ears in the same manner as you did with the sideburns. Hold the hair upward and, pulling down as you work your way towards the top of the head, work with the right side of the head first and then the left. Again, it is worth noting that if you always work in the same manner, there is never a question as to whether you checked that area yet or not.

Keep in mind that your approach depends solely on the length of hair you are examining. Generally hair 2" or shorter will be fanned, while hair longer than 2" (yet still too short to grasp all at once) is easier if held in sections. One exception to that rule is hair that is at or just above shoulder length, typical of a short-haired girl. In such cases we prefer to split the hair down the middle, clasping one half up while working our imaginary ponytail (or in this case, pigtail) technique on the first side, and then repeat the process on the other side. If the hair style is one which is long on the sides and short at the nape of the neck, blend these techniques in order to thoroughly examine all of the hair.

Now that you have completed the manual exam, follow up with a good **comb-out**. Hand a paper towel to the individual you are checking, have them cover their eyes and ask them to tilt their head back. With their head tilted, lightly spray mint spritz around the hair, being careful to avoid the eye area. If you do not have a mint spritz or other safe solution, dry comb the hair. Use a good lice comb for two to three minutes, and comb starting at the scalp and working to the ends of the hair. Remember to comb at a 90-degree angle to increase the odds of uncovering potential **evidence**. This process should be repeated in multiple directions--backward, downward, and upward motions--always starting at the root of the hair and working all the way to the end. During **comb-out**, check the comb often for **evidence**. Again, if **evidence** is found **at any time**, STOP! **Treatment** is now needed.

Assuming no **evidence** is found you can now comb the hair back with a detangler comb and put your tools away until the next **head check**.

"THE SHEPHERD METHOD™"

(Treatment Process)

Tools Used: detangler comb, quality lice comb; non-toxic lice shampoo; mousse or other safe, alternative product; duck clips; wooden stick; tissue or paper towels; water bucket (not all of these tools may be needed). To purchase needed items, check your local pharmacy, beauty supply store or visit: www.licesloutions.org.

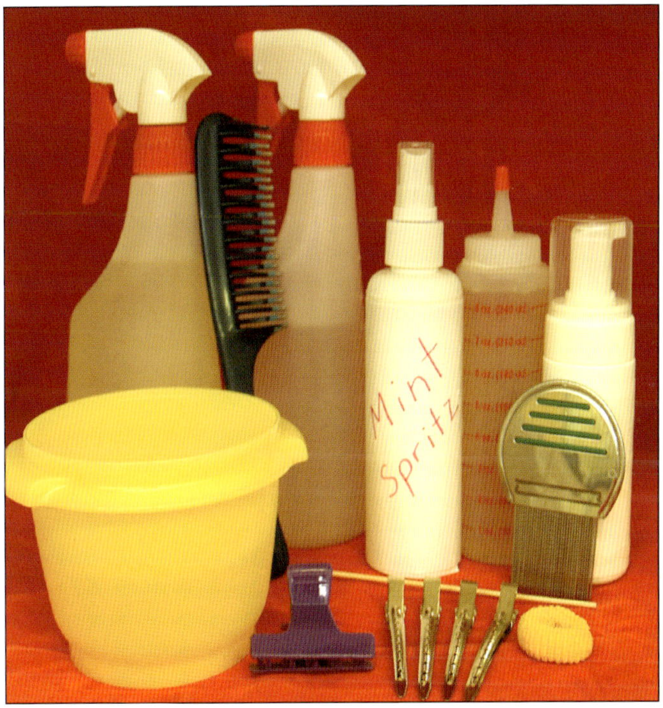

It is advisable to have your tools ready before starting the treatment process. Suggested tools might include: Treatment product of your choice, detangler comb, quality lice comb, hair clips, duck clips, hair ties, wooden stick, bucket of water, spray bottle of water and mint spritz.

*{Always confirm **evidence** of head lice prior to any **treatment**.}*

*<u>**Evidence** is considered to be either nits or bugs.</u>*

A Treatment Process consists of the following steps:

Prepare tools for easy access during the **treatment** process. This should include a bucket of water in which you can rinse the comb and place the bugs as you work your way through the hair.

Using a detangler comb, comb the hair free of tangles. Ensuring that the hair is tangle-free will make the caregiver's job easier and is more comfortable for the individual.

Provide a paper towel to the individual being treated and ask them to cover their eyes. Be careful that their head is tipped back before applying product to their hair. Doing so will reduce the risk of the product running into their eyes. Exercise caution when applying product not to over-saturate the hair. It should be just damp enough (similar to towel-dried hair) to glide the lice comb through easily. It is far easier to work with hair that is <u>not</u> over-saturated. Hair should be just wet enough to cause a

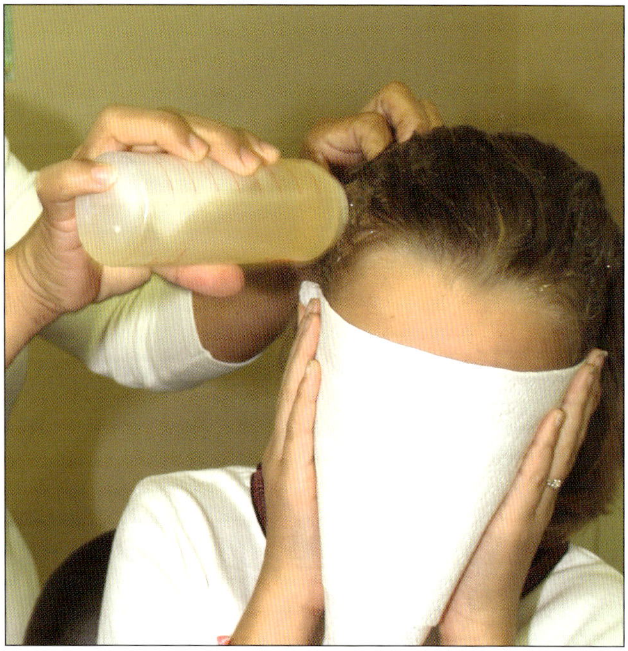

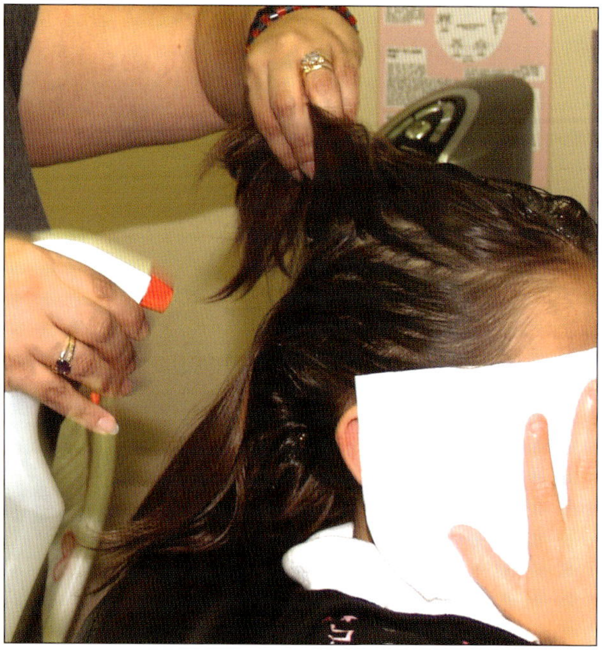

As you apply treatment product be careful to wet all hair, while not over saturating it. Always protect the eyes! Left: Apply product around the hair line. Right: Lifting hair and spraying product throughout allows for a more complete coverage.

slick surface, allowing for an aggressive and thorough **comb-out**. Additional product can be applied to hair as it begins to dry out. Any remaining product could also be added during the **final re-check.** I have found that too much product complicates the **treatment process.**

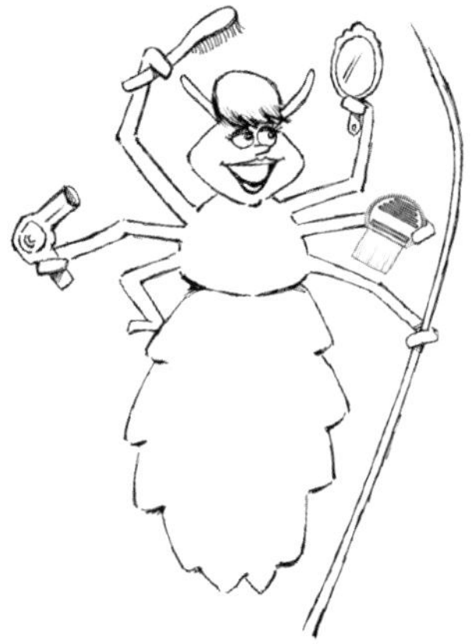

> Just a pesky reminder: protect the individual's eyes while applying any product and ensure that their head is tilted back.

As you move into the actual separation of the hair and **strand-by-strand** nit removal, the process will be far more successful if the hair is <u>not</u> dripping wet. Once you have applied product, comb hair completely until the lice comb is coming up clean. Next, divide hair into three sections and secure it, leaving only Section One down to work with. If the section you are working on is over-saturated, use a hand towel or paper towel to wring out excess liquid. Once the excess product has been removed, you can move more efficiently through the hair.

<u>Lice comb</u>: Using a good lice comb, begin with what we refer to as an **initial comb-out**. Done properly, this will remove at least 85% of the individual's nit and bug load. A good **initial comb-out** is in your best interest as it helps minimize the actual time needed to manually pick nits. A good rule of thumb is 20 swipes with no further **evidence** removed. When **combing out**, position the lice comb against the scalp, resting the teeth of the comb gently on the surface of the scalp. Be careful

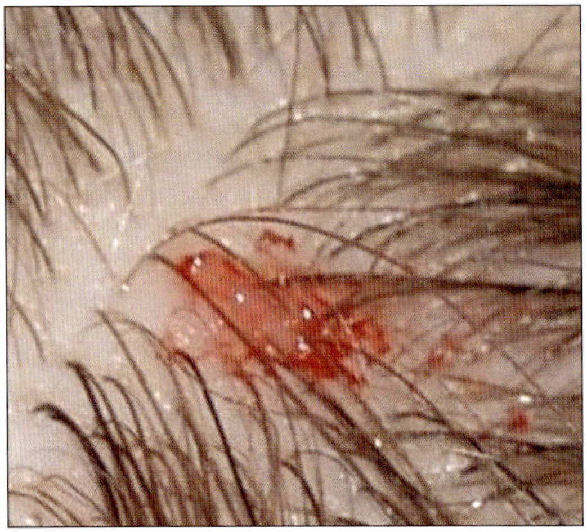

Open sores from scratching can lead to secondary infections

not to allow teeth to dig into the head or cause abrasions. We often see children who have tread marks on their scalp. This is not only unnecessary but is also dangerous, as it could lead to secondary infections.

Please Note: Head lice do not burrow, they live on the surface of your scalp. Comb the hair starting at the roots and working from the scalp all the way to the end of the hair shaft. It is important that you not stop the combing process midway, as this could allow bugs an opportunity to escape. Repeat the process in multiple directions--combing the hair in backward, downward, and upward motions. While you are doing the **initial combing out**, rinse the comb in the water bucket as necessary to remove excessive nits or any time a bug has been captured in the comb. It is not necessary to rinse the comb with each swipe, as nits cannot reattach themselves. However, as you collect them on the comb or any time you remove

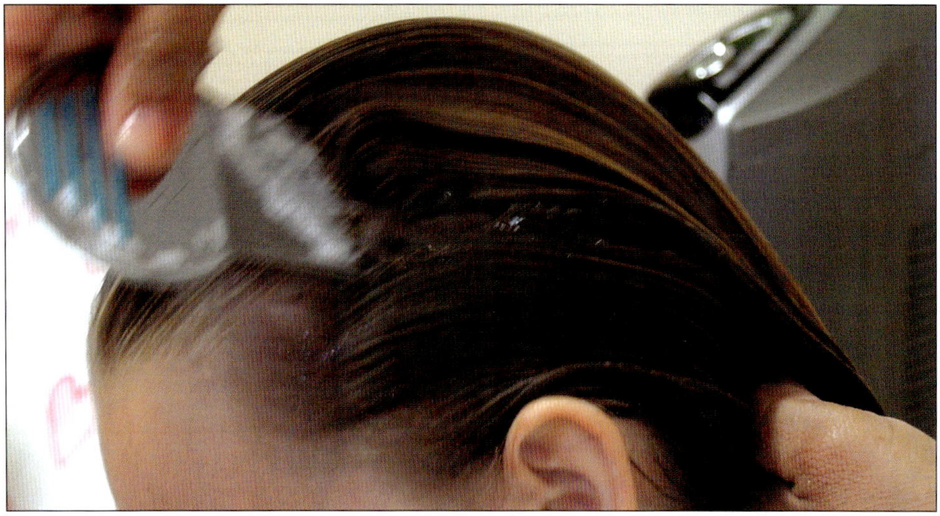

A thorough **initial comb-out** done with a quality lice comb can remove at least 85% of nits and bugs in an individual's head of hair.

a bug, it is advisable to rinse the comb at that time. Continue combing in this manner with the lice comb until you are no longer seeing any **evidence** of lice or nits on the comb. Again, the more **evidence** you remove now, the less time you will have to spend picking nits.

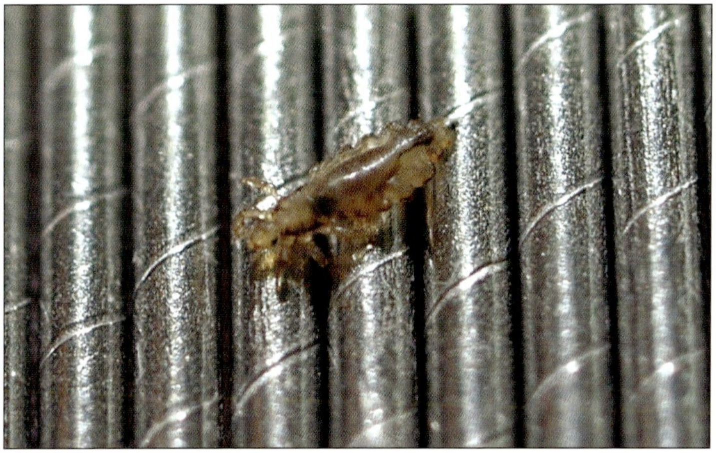

Remember to check the comb for **evidence** of lice, and properly dispose of any bugs removed.

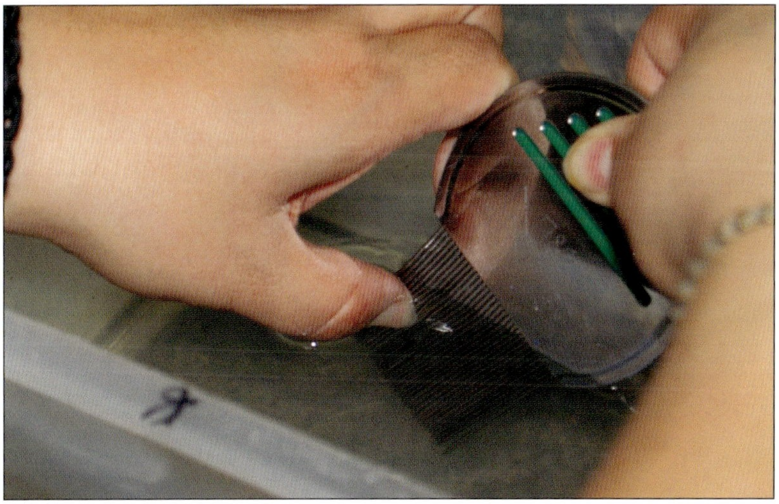

Fanning the teeth of your lice comb in the bucket of water will help remove lice and nits.

This should take approximately 15 to 30 minutes, depending upon the severity of the infestation and thickness of the individual's hair. Keep in mind this is not intended to remove everything. However, a good **initial comb-out** will reduce overall **nit picking** time and ensure greater success upon completion of the **treatment**. It is further recommended that you take a minute to re-comb each section as you begin to work in that area, as bugs will constantly try to move away from you. Don't be surprised if you find additional lice in Section Four, as this is the last section you will work with.

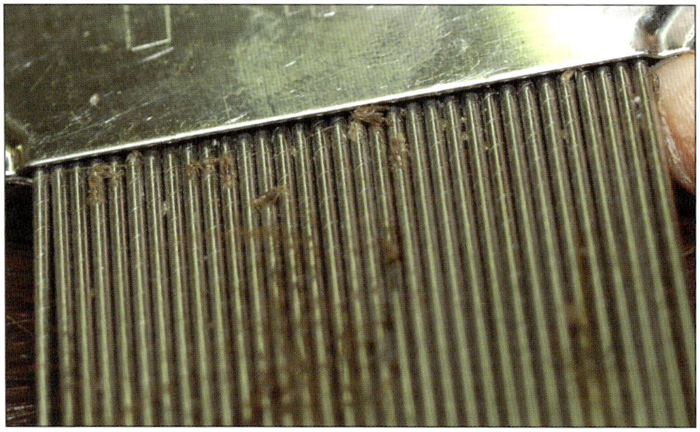

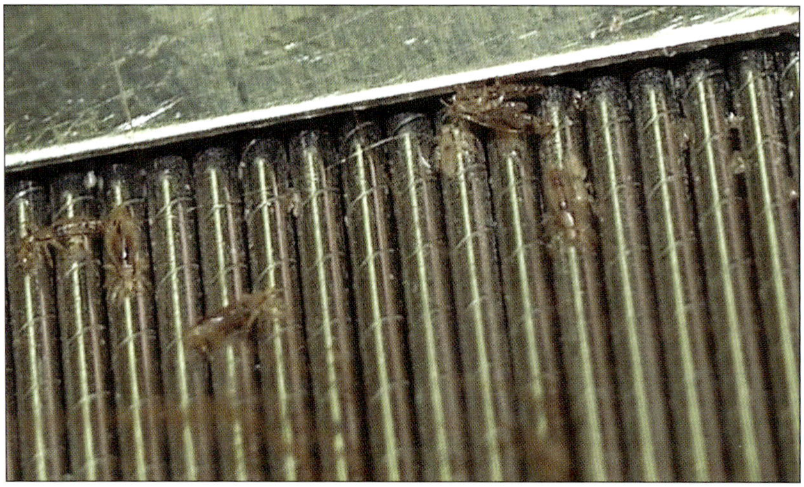

Lice and nits are easily identifiable on the teeth of a good lice comb. This enlarged view shows numerous lice combed out in just one swipe.

By far, the most critical part of the **treatment process** is the actual nit removal process. To ensure absolute success, the caregiver must diligently, painstakingly and tediously remove all the nits and bugs from the individual's hair and head. Keep in mind that this is a time-consuming process and there are <u>no</u> shortcuts for doing the job right. It is essential that the caregiver work in paper-thin layers of hair as they make their way through the hair - and I mean as thin as a piece of paper. Working with a thicker layer will speed up the process but also offers an opportunity for bugs to hide. Additionally, since nits are attached only to one side of the hair shaft, it is imperative to work with paper thin layers to ensure you are not missing nits between the layers.

> "Did you ever wonder where the phrase "nit picking" came from? Now you know, it refers to the tedious process of picking lice eggs from someone's hair."

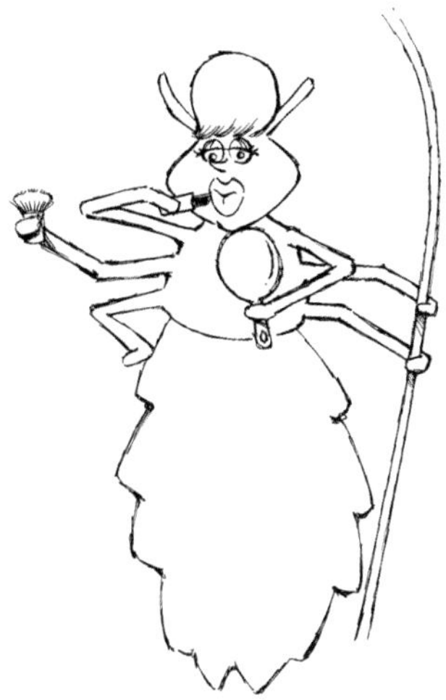

Next you are ready to **nit pick**. Begin by sectioning the hair. Rather than parting down the middle of the head, I prefer, for several reasons, a more asymmetrical parting of the hairs, which allows a larger amount of hair to be on the right side of the head while leaving less hair on the left. Bugs tend to congregate along the very top of the head. By allowing that slight overlap of the middle part, I am giving the bugs a false sense of security. The end result is less scattering of the bugs, particularly where the nymphs are concerned, and it increases my odds of finding them in the process. Additionally, by starting with a larger portion of hair, we reduce the time necessary on Sections 3 and 4. Since your treatment subject (especially if they are a child) may tend to get impatient, this allows the final sections to progress more quickly.

It is important to keep your lines as straight as possible while maintaining paper thin layers. Attention to this detail ensures greater success in your quest for lice and nits. Using a detangler comb, part the hair one to two inches to the left side of the midline. Next, secure the left side of the hair, separating it from the right side, by twisting the left side into one large bun. These will eventually

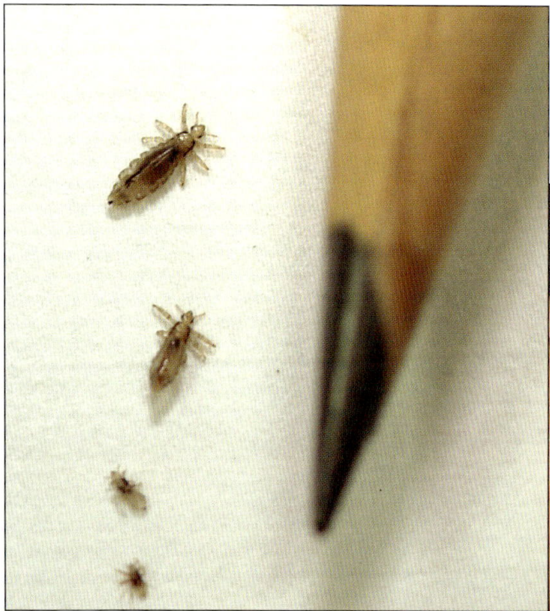

From top to bottom is an adult louse, 3rd, 2nd, and 1st stage nymphs.

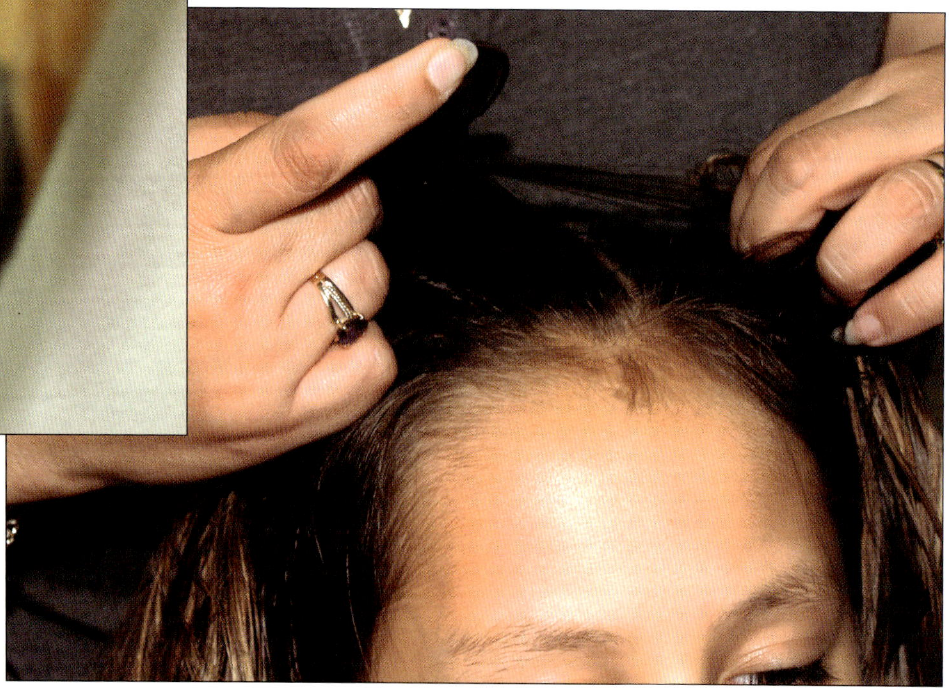

Before starting to "nit-pick", separate hair into sections. The hair should be parted to the left side of the mid-line of the head.

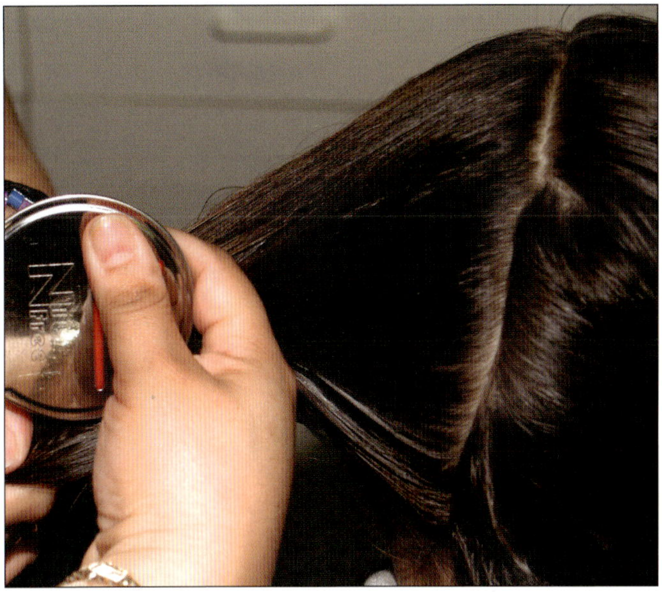

Comb through hair and then twist the left side of the hair into a bun. This will later become Sections 3 and 4.

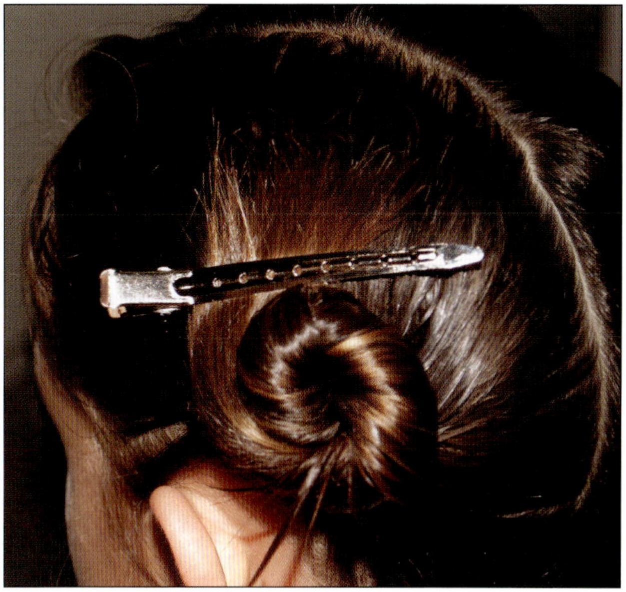

A large duck clip helps hold the hair securely out of your way until you are ready to work in that section.

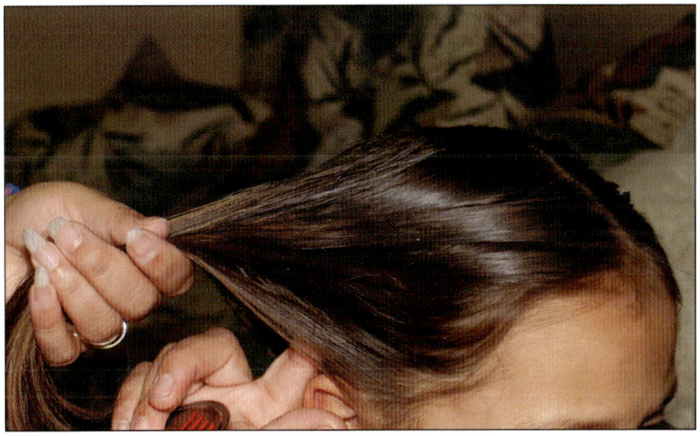

Divide the hair in half just behind the ear. The hair to the front of the ear is Section 1, while the hair behind the ear is Section 2.

become Sections 3 and 4. Now, part the right side of the hair in half into Sections 1 and 2. This is done by using the detangler comb to part hair beginning from the top of the head, moving straight down to the area just above the back side of the ear. Section 1 is the area in front of the ear, while Section 2 is the area behind the ear. Twist Section 2 into a tight bun using duck clips, securing the hair tightly. Only the section you are currently working on will be loose, while the remaining three sections should be secured in tight buns. This will hold true as

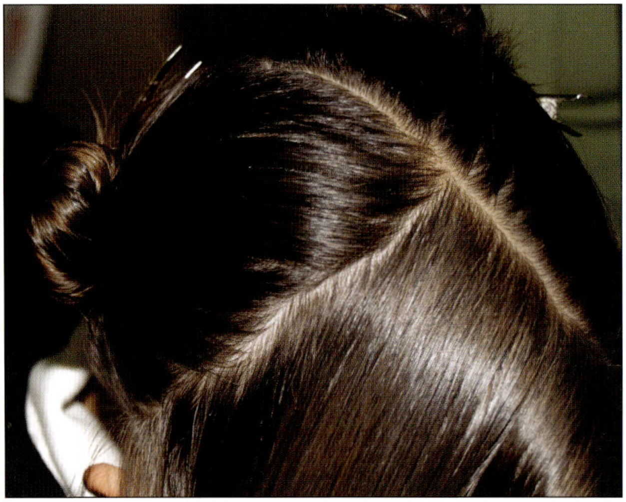

Only the section you are working on should be loose. Pictured above you can see that the right front, or Section 1, is loose while Section 2 is in a tight bun waiting its turn to be treated.

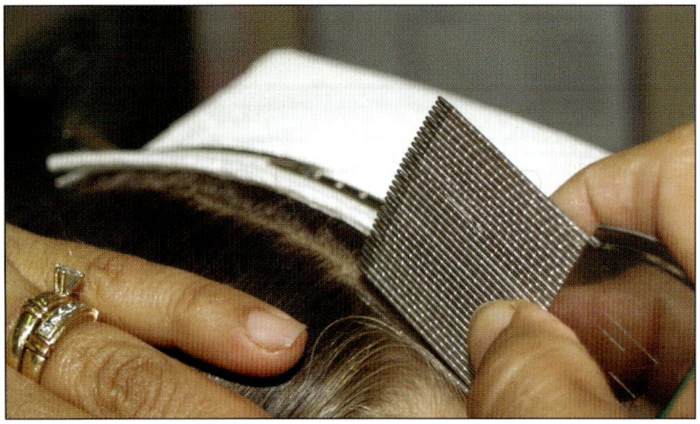

Note that the hair has been properly secured and a tissue has been placed over Sections 3 and 4 allowing you a clean surface to work with. Clip each clean layer out of the way as you work your way through the section.

you work your way through the hair, no matter what section you are working on.

Before you begin your lice removal process, cover the left side of the head with a paper towel. Duck clips will help hold the towel securely in place. This is done to allow for a clean surface onto which the caregiver can flip clean hairs as they work their way through the right side of the head. As you begin your nit-picking and lice-combing process, start at Section 1 (right front side of head).

Nit-picking Technique: Begin at the top of the head (at the mid-line, the parted area you created) and work in a horizontal motion. You can use the nail on your index finger, a wooden stick or tooth of a comb to separate the hair in a straight, paper-thin layer. (Keep in mind this is a personal preference and makes no difference as long as you are able to work efficiently and keep your lines straight.) You should then work your way through each layer with the lice comb. Be careful to closely examine the hair as well as the scalp. Nits tend to be reflective, which is why it is advisable to check the head in a well-lit area or the natural light of outdoors. The bugs, on the other hand, are like chameleons and can blend

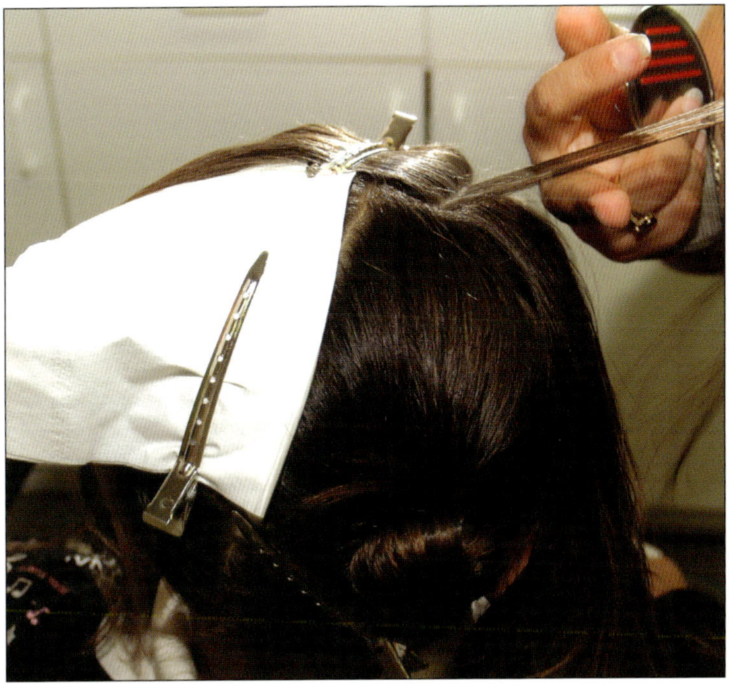

Note that the hair has been properly secured and a tissue placed over Sections 3 and 4 allowing you a clean surface to work with. Clip each clean layer out of the way as you work your way through the section.

with their environment. It is not uncommon to look right at a bug and not even see it. A trick of the trade is the fact that they cannot camouflage their intestinal tract. Therefore, you'll see what appears to be a speck of dirt or a freckle on the scalp. Anytime you see this, tap it with your fingernail, comb or wooden stick. If it takes off running, it is a bug! Generally the easiest way to remove the bug is to slide the teeth of your lice comb under the bug and slowly glide the comb all the way down the hair shaft and off the head! Some people prefer to grab the bug with their nails. That is fine if you have the proper nails to do it. However, in doing so be extra careful to get the bug off your nails and into the bucket to prevent infesting yourself.

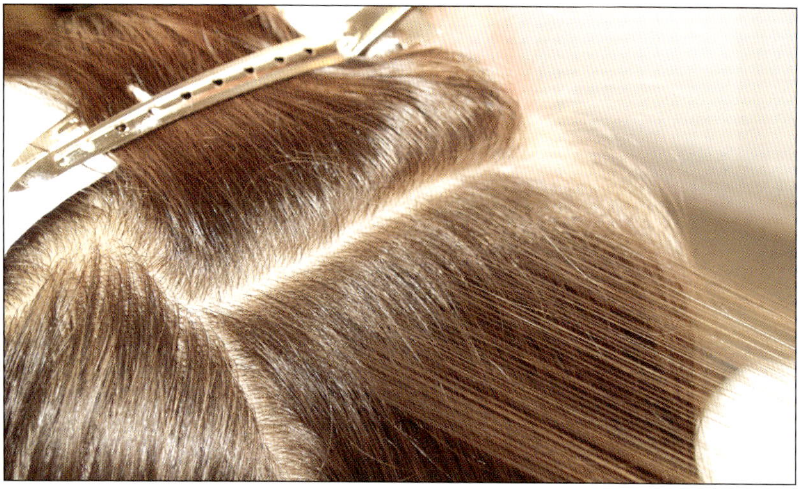

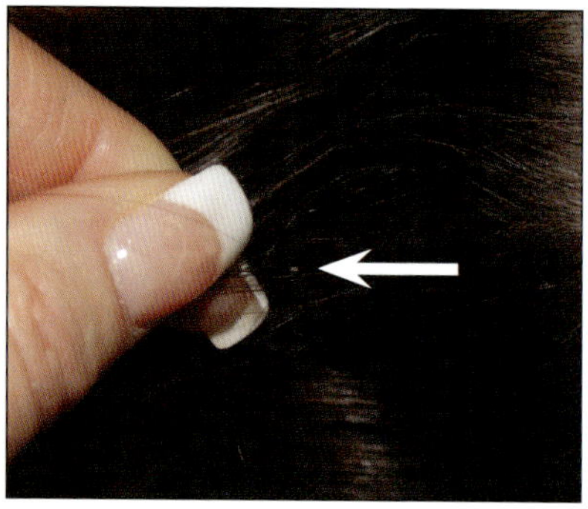

Left: By working in paper thin layers you are able to inspect the scalp as well as all strands of hair.

Right: Finding every nit is a tedious and time consuming process but well worth it when you have a successful treatment the first time.

Finding a nit on the hair is like looking for a needle in a haystack. Therefore, you must be aggressive in your approach. We check, **re-check**, and triple-check not only our own work but each other's as well. Our goal, as should be yours, is to do the job right the first time so that it is not necessary to put the child or yourself through multiple time-consuming **treatments**. Treat once and keep **re-checking** to ensure that nothing has been missed and no further contact exits.

Now that you have combed the hair and examined the scalp, take your fingers in a scissor-like motion and run them along the same layer of hair. As before, start at the root of hair and feel all the way to the end of the hair shaft. If the hair is paper-thin and a nit does exist, you will feel it. The best description I can offer is that it feels like you are driving a car over a speed bump. If you feel a nit, you must search further until you find and remove it.

Finally, and this is a very important part of the process, take your free hand and hold it under the section of the hair that you just worked on. A nit that might be invisible as you look through the hair will stand out when placed next to the shaded contrast of your hand. To further exemplify this, we like to share the following example. When we treat in our office, we rinse our lice combs in a clear bucket of water. When we invite parents to peek in the bucket to see what we combed out, they are

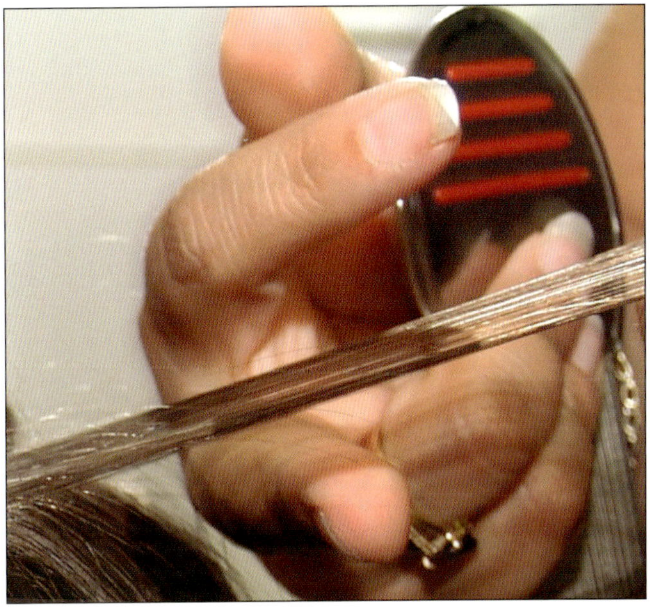

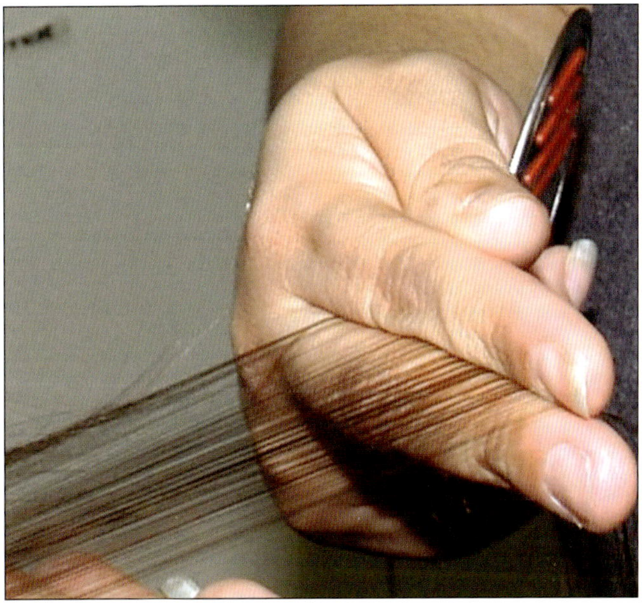

Placing a finger on either side of the hair and moving along the layer in a scissor like motion will enable you to feel any nits that you might not otherwise have seen. A nit on the hair feels much like a car driving over a speed bump.

usually amazed to observe all the bugs that were in their child's hair. However, if we hold the bucket suspended in the air and ask them to look into it, they barely see what we collected. Why? Because instead of looking in the bucket they are looking through it. The same holds true with the hair. By holding it out with nothing to shade it, the very thing you are looking for will seemingly disappear. This is another trick of the trade that is an important step towards total eradication.

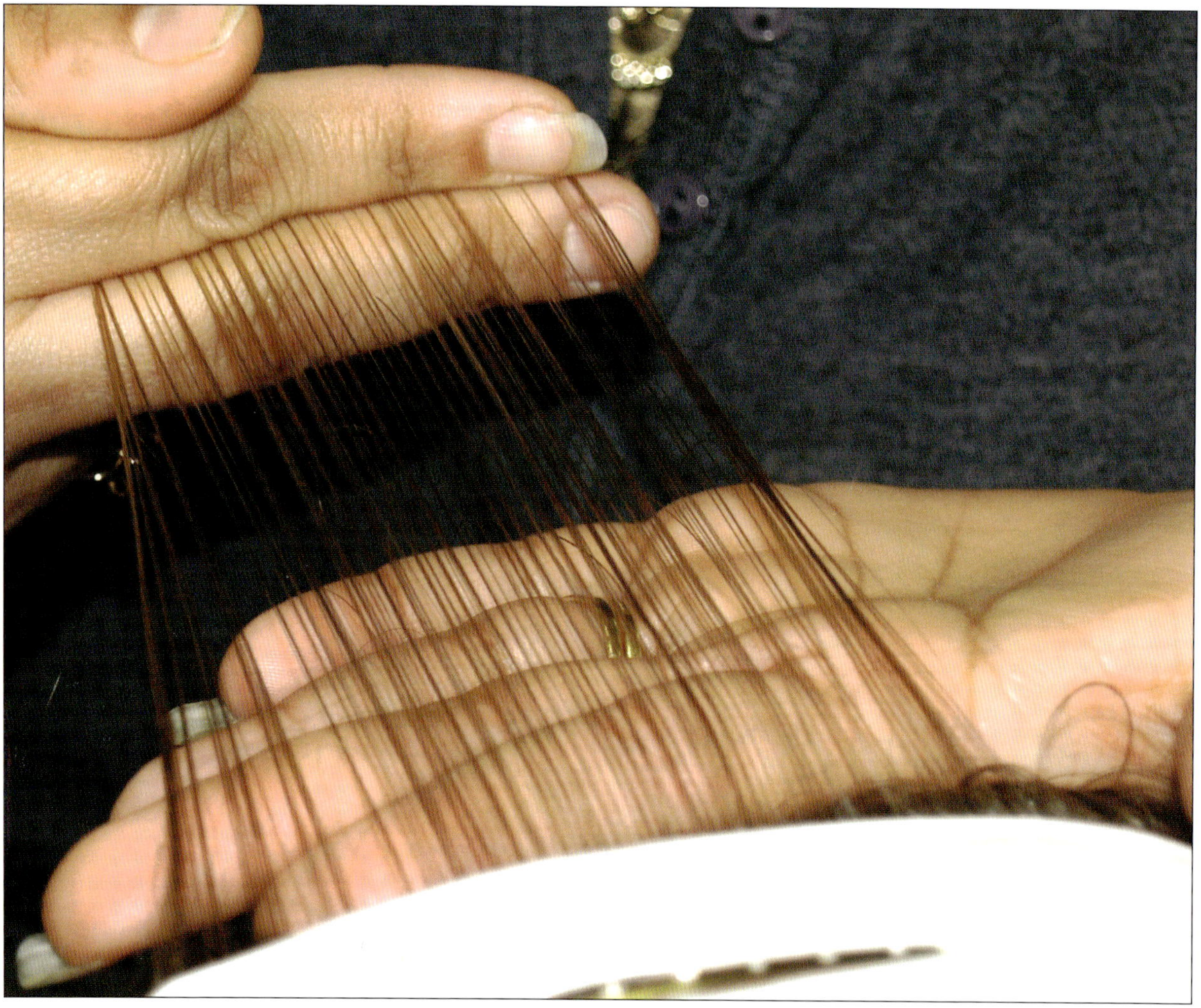

Shown is the technician shading the hair with her left hand and using a scissor-like motion with her right hand.

So what if you do find a nit? First, don't panic or stress--your goal is to find any remaining nits. Removing nits is easy. Simply take your fingernails and slide the nit down to the end of the hair (be sure to go **all** the way to the end of the strand of hair). Eggs or nits are attached by a fixative glue which the bug secretes as she lays the egg. This glue is so fast-drying that the female louse has on rare occasions been known to glue herself to the hair. The glue is similar to very strong cement and can be difficult to remove as you attempt to glide the nit down the hair. It is not uncommon to think you pulled the nit off, only to see it still on the hair. Therefore, make sure that the nit was removed by looking for it on your fingers. Off the hair the nit is of no danger because it cannot reattach itself.

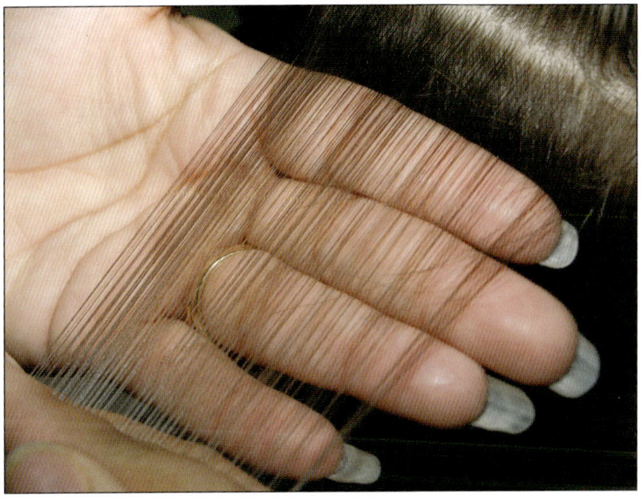

Shading is vital to ensure you find all the nits.

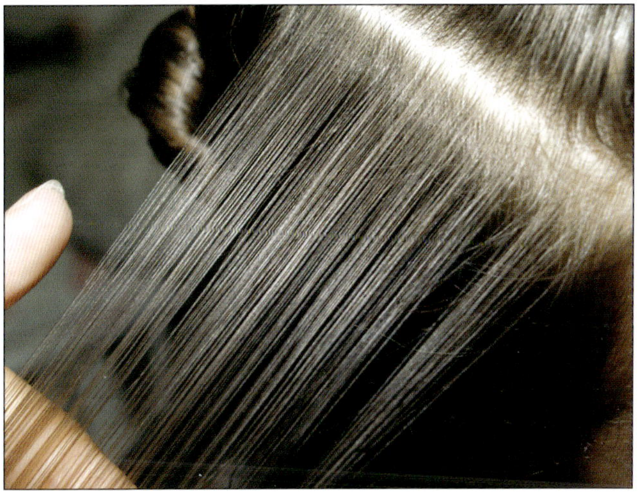

Don't forget to keep the lines straight, layers thin, and gently but securely hold the hair away from the scalp area as you examine each layer.

Unlike the bugs, which should be placed into water, you can drop nits on the floor for later cleanup. Be assured that once separated from the head, it is highly unlikely that the nit will hatch, as it needs the warmth of the body to incubate (much like a chicken sitting on an egg). Another fact worth noting is that a nit off the hair resembles a tiny tadpole. What appears to be a tail is actually the glue that came off with the egg. We often hear about parents who choose to cut the nit out rather than remove it with their nails. While that might seem like the easiest and fastest way of doing it, in many cases, the child could have such a severe infestation that this sort of removal process would leave them with not only a bad haircut, but very little hair.

Don't forget to carefully examine the scalp as you work your way through each paper-thin layer of hair. Newly hatched lice, or nymphs, live directly on the scalp and look like specks of dirt on the head. If you think you see what appears to be a speck of dirt or freckle, tap it. If it takes off running, it is a bug. I believe that one of the biggest reasons parents struggle to get past head lice is because they fail to recognize the nymphs. Much emphasis is placed on the importance of removing all the nits, but very little is said about the nymphs. Unlike nits that may or may not be viable, every nymph you

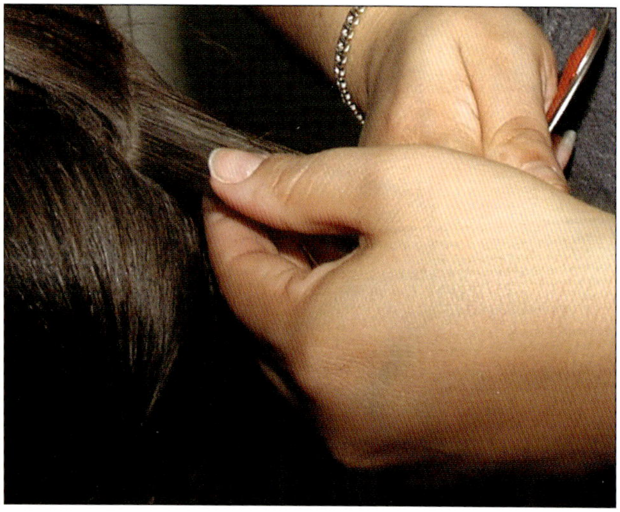

Technician removes a nit with her fingers.

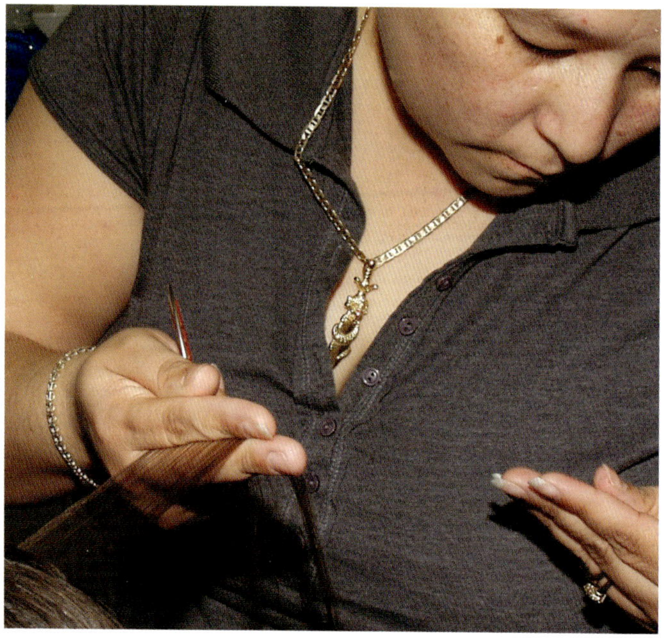

While still supporting the layer of hair, the technician examines her fingers to make certain the nit was removed.

remove is a living, breathing parasite just waiting to start its own family. Nymphs come in three sizes: first stage, second stage, and third stage. Newer terminology refers to them as "instar," rather than stages. Regardless of what you call them, they are very difficult to remove and even more difficult to find. When I speak publicly, I always tell the audience to imagine they are holding a pencil that is sharpened to a very fine point. That point is how tiny a newly hatched nymph is and one of the primary reasons it is so difficult to remove.

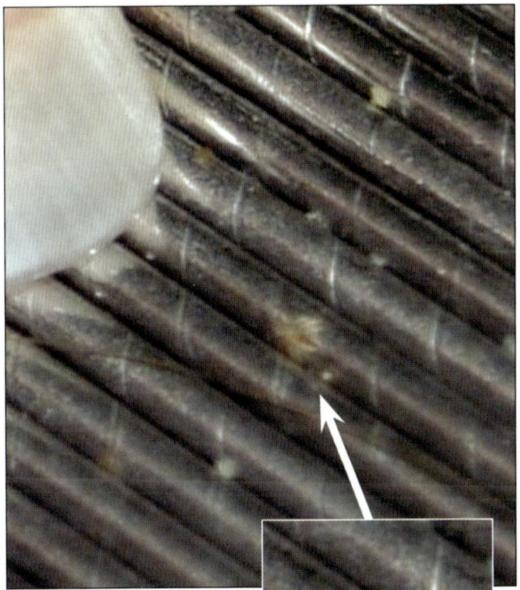

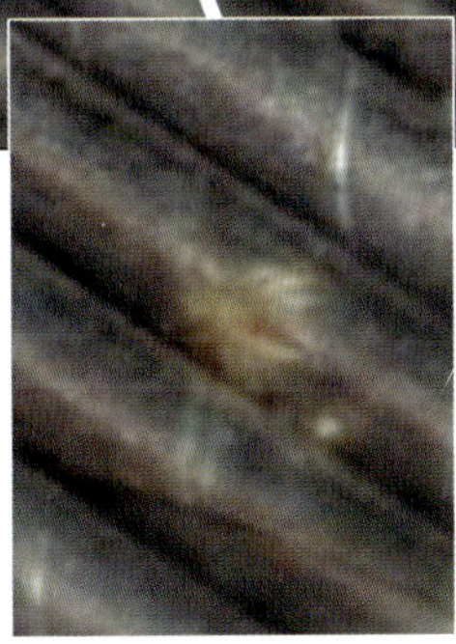

Although the nymph is extremely small, it is still visible on the teeth of the comb.

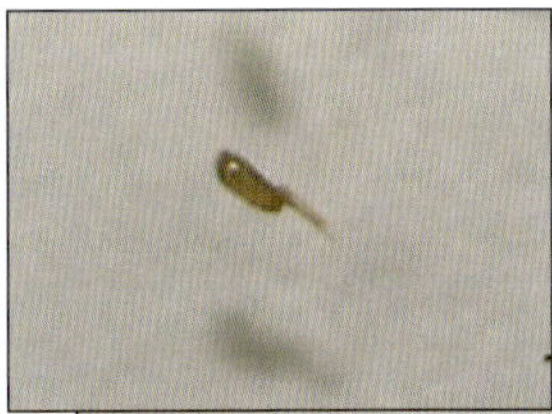

It's easy to see the tadpole appearance in this enlarged photo.

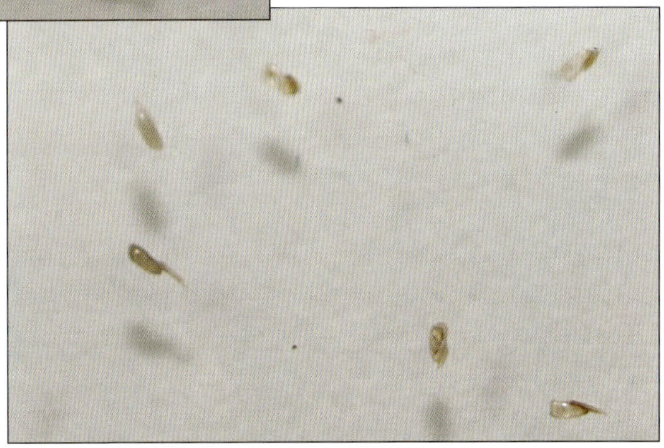

This picture shows several nits that were combed off an individual's hair. Off the hair they take on a tadpole appearance. What looks like the tail is actually the fixative glue that remains attached to the nit even after the nit has been removed from the hair.

There is no right or wrong way to remove the nymph, as long as in the end they are removed. Only you can decide what works best for you. Many lice technicians prefer to just grab them with their fingernails. This is fine if you have the nails to work with or if the nymph does not disappear into other parts of the hair. Another way, and the one I generally prefer, is to place the teeth of the comb under the moving bug, securing the bug on the teeth, and then comb it out to the end of the hair. Make certain that the nymph is in fact on the teeth of the comb. If not, it is imperative to continue combing the area until you come up with the bug.

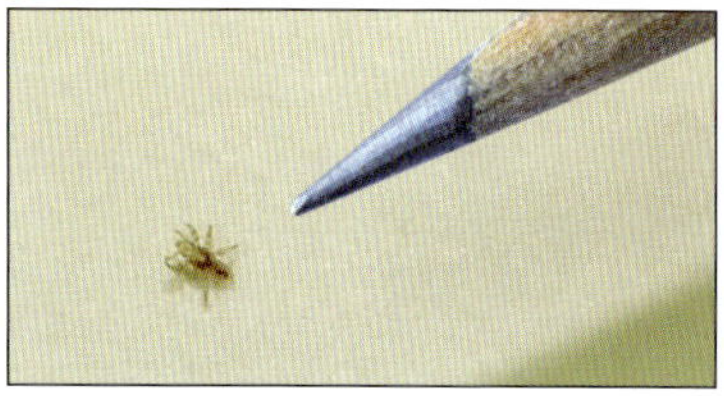

The smallest of nymphs is no bigger than the tip of a very sharp pencil.

At no time should you move on with the **treatment** without first removing a known nymph. While it may take extra time and patience to remove the nymph, it is time well spent. As hard as nymphs are to remove, they are even more difficult to spot in the first place. If you see a nymph, don't risk thinking you'll get it out later. Always take the time to get them out when you first see them. Leaving bugs (or in this case nymphs) behind is asking for trouble. I can't emphasize enough the importance of doing it right the first time, so you don't have to do it again and again.

OK, so you are going through the head, find a nymph along the way and remove the bug. Then what? Dispose of it properly. As I explained earlier, in our office we keep a clear bucket of water at each of the technician's stations. When we find a bug on the head, regardless of whether it is a first-stage nymph or an adult louse, we always dispose of it in the bucket. The biggest concern for me is that it has been disposed of. Why? If the bug is left on the comb, there is the risk of giving it a free ride back into the head of hair being treated. If you remove it with your hand and fail to make certain that it is placed in the bucket, there is always the risk that you could inadvertently infest yourself, now becoming the individual in need of a **treatment**. It's my experience that one-third of mothers treating their infested child end up having lice as well. Although close contact accounts for some instances of transfer, many cases occur as a result of careless **treatment** processes. When it comes to **treatments** our motto is, "Always stay to the side of caution and be safe in everything you do."

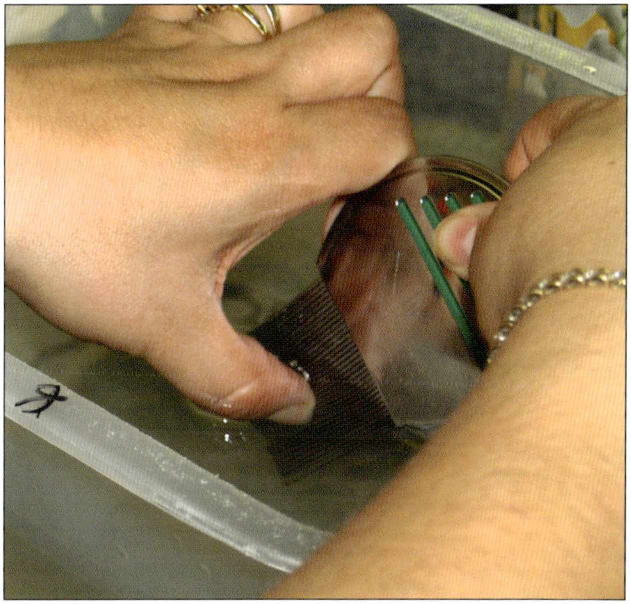

Disposing of bugs properly prevents unnecessary transmission.

As you work through each layer of hair, flip the clean and examined layer of hair onto the left side and clip it down with a duck clip, being careful to keep clean strands separated from hair that has not yet been examined. (Your tissue separation is sufficient, as bugs will primarily be close to the scalp. Keep in mind you will still be doing a **final re-check** on completion, so don't let this part over-stress you.) Continue this process all the way to the bottom of Section 1. Be extra careful with baby-fine strands around the ear area, as this is a popular place for lice to lay eggs. Once completed, tie Section 1 into a tight bun and let down Section 2.

Repeat the previous process as you begin to work with Section 2. Take the lice comb and comb thoroughly through this section. Again, if you remove additional bugs, carefully dispose of them in your water bucket. Repeating the process done in Section 1, comb again, working from the top of the head to the bottom in thin, horizontal layers. Hairs in this area should be flipped up and around the bun on Section 1 and clipped tightly as you move through this section of hair. Since Section 1 has been cleaned and examined, there is no risk in the hairs (of Sections 1 and 2) having contact with each other. As always, be extra careful to examine the fine, newly grown hairs around the nape of the neck (including any indented area at the base of the skull), as this is another popular place for lice to hide their nits. When this area is complete, tie the hair back into a bun and secure it tightly.

Moving now onto the left side, remove the tissue or paper towel from the individual's head. Hair which was initially placed into one large bun should now be separated into two smaller halves, providing you with the area in front of the ear as Section 3 and the area behind the ear as Section 4. Tie Section 4 back into a bun and begin working on Section 3. Remember, this will be the area on the left side of the head and in front of the ear. **Comb out** the entire section before proceeding with the **strand-by-strand** removal.

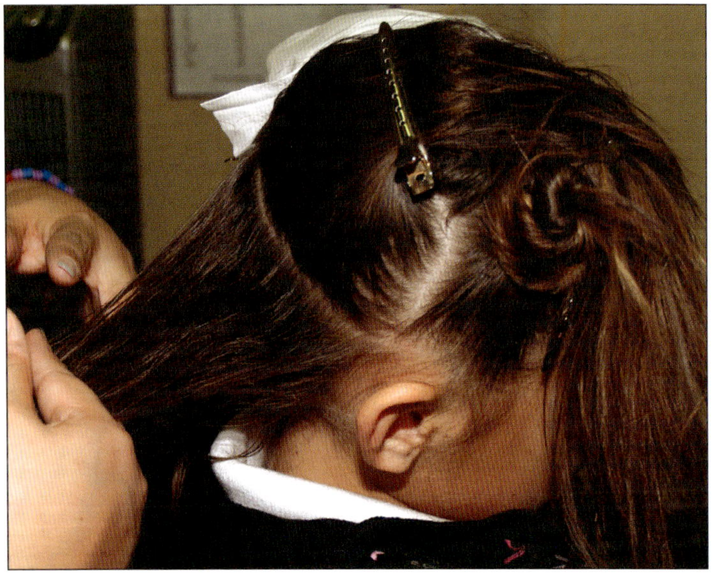

The technician has advanced to Section 2 and is now flipping the examined hair around the tight bun of Section 1.

When a good **comb-out** of this section is completed, repeat the process of working your way through the hair, as was done on Sections 1 and 2. However, you will now be flipping and clipping hair onto Section 1. You don't need a paper towel or divider at this time, as the hair you are flipping layers onto has already been examined. Be careful as you work your way through the hair to examine both the hair and the scalp, removing any **evidence** you might find.

Although you may be getting tired at this point, and the individual you are treating might be getting impatient, don't rush the process. Be as thorough as possible <u>every</u> step of the way. It's perfectly acceptable to take a break at any time, as long as you secure the hair (keeping the treated hair away from hair not yet treated) and complete the process immediately following a few moments of rest. Tie Section 3 in a bun once you've completed examining that area. Closely examine baby-fine hairs around the bottom of each section. We prefer to give these hairs an extra going-over upon completion just to be safe. Remain mindful that many newly-laid nits are extremely close to the root of the hair, often appearing to be part of that root. That is one of the many reasons that you can look for days, not seeing a thing, and then with a little hair growth notice a nit.

Having completed Sections 1 and 2, separate hair on left side of head creating Sections 3 and 4.

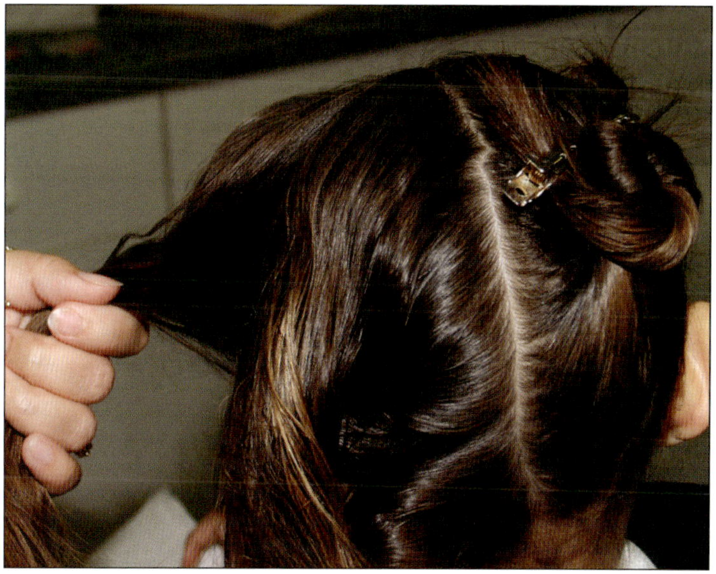

As you move on to your final section, begin by releasing the hair in Section 4. As you did in the previous three sections, comb through this section prior to working in paper-thin layers. This is extremely important, as the bugs will always be moving away from where you are working. As you systematically make your way through the hair, you force them into the last section, allowing you to capture many of them in the process. Section 4 will be completed in the same manner as previous sections. Be careful to work in PAPER-THIN layers as you comb, examine, feel and shade each layer of hair. If the individual has bangs, that area should be treated last and in the same manner recommended in the head check section, working from the forehead back. Examine the area carefully, as it is not uncommon to find numerous nits in this area.

Congratulations, you've completed your strand-by-strand inspection and are ready to start your **final re-check**. In order to assure an accurate inspection of the hair, blow it dry. While it's far easier to treat wet hair, it is much easier to examine a dry head of hair.

From a professional standpoint, we prefer to bring in a second set of eyes for this process. Our most skilled technicians perform this task. Having a second person walk through the process of a **final re-check** ensures that everything was removed. If you are working with someone else, treating one child at a time, I suggest you flip caregivers for this portion of the **treatment process**. If you are working alone, it is all right to check your own work, but do so slowly and methodically, carefully looking for anything you might have missed.

The **final re-check** is very similar to the **initial head check**, only in thinner layers, and you will be removing additional **evidence** you find along the way. For individuals with longer hair, secure the hair with one hand and position it high on the head as in an imaginary ponytail. Keep in mind the caregiver will be holding the hair in this manner during the entire **re-check** process. Using your free hand, pull down thin layers of hair with either a wooden stick or your fingernail (this is a personal preference). If you find additional **evidence**, don't get discouraged. It's "easier to treat wet hair, easier to see on dry hair." That is why you cannot afford to skip this phase of the process, no matter how tired you are. If the individual being treated needs to take a break or stretch, now would be a good time, as long as they return to you after a short break to complete the **final re-check**. If you find further **evidence**, remove it, being careful to dispose of bugs into your water bucket.

As was done with the **initial head check**, the caregiver should begin pulling thin layers of hair from the bottom of the neck area, around the ears, and sideburns. Always pull thin layers from side to side, evenly moving upward around the head. As mentioned in the part on Section 4, if bugs exist they will be moving away from you. In this case, they are moving up. Therefore, once you reach the top of the head, an additional **comb-out** along the midline area is necessary. By checking the hair in this manner, you now see the hairs from a different angle, increasing opportunities to identify missed nits. As the caregiver works their way through the hair, they must examine the scalp area as well. Lice are like chameleons and can blend in with their environment, effectively camouflaging their entire bodies, with the exception of their intestinal tracts. While the outer shell of the body can appear totally opaque, the intestinal tract remains dark. This is why looking for what appears to be a dark speck of dirt is so important. If you see a dark speck, tap it; if it takes off running, it is a bug! If the individual you are treating has extremely thick hair, it's advisable to do a few extra comb-throughs as you work your way to the top of the head. By doing this you are able to comb areas that would otherwise be buried in the depths of the hair. Be absolutely certain to comb all the way to the end of the hair.

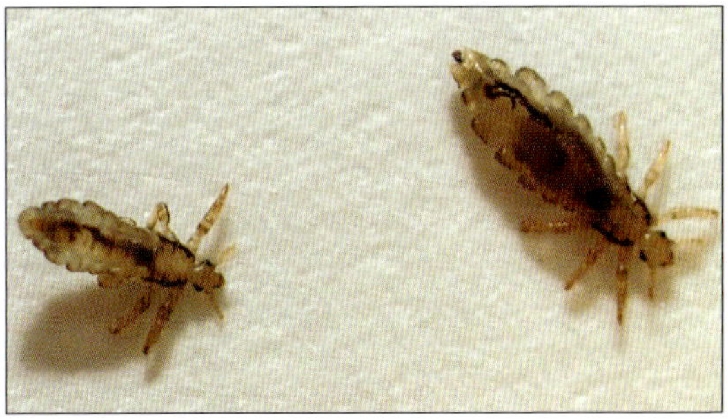

The outer shell of the body can appear totally opaque while the intestinal tract remains dark.

Once you reach the top of the head, re-comb the area that makes up one inch from each side of the middle of the head. This leaves you with approximately a 2" width of hair (the approximate depth of a decent lice comb).

Holding the hair securely at the top, use the lice comb. Holding it against the scalp, go into the middle of your 2" wide section and comb, moving up all the way to the ends of the hair. Be sure to comb the entire area in this manner, working from all directions, basically combing in a complete circle. It is not unusual to find several bugs in this final step, as their goal is to survive the **treatment process,** while yours is to eliminate them. Combing them out now makes the examination of the last hairs easier and far more successful. If you find bugs, don't be alarmed, just remove them and dispose of them into the water bucket. Continue combing until all of the upper area is combed through and you find no further **evidence.** After completing the **comb-out** on the top of the head, continue pulling the last of the thin layers until there are no more layers to be checked. If the individual has bangs, it is now time to check them. Hold the bangs up with one hand or simply push them back, holding them down in the process. Start checking the bangs by pulling thin layers down at the forehead, working your way back until all the bangs have been examined.

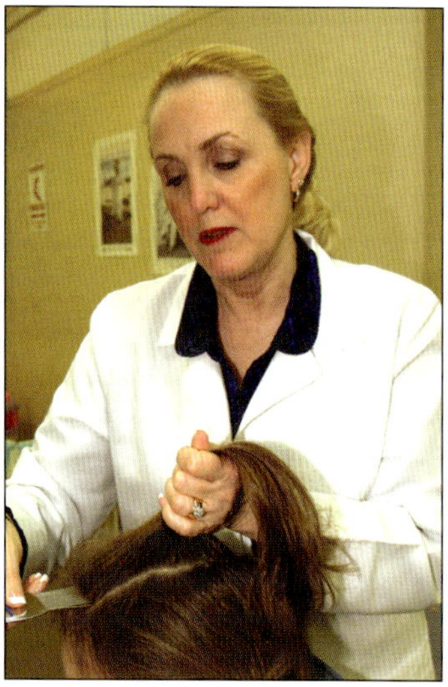

During the **Final Recheck**, it is important to take extra time and care along the top of the head, by combing approximately one inch to each side of the middle part.

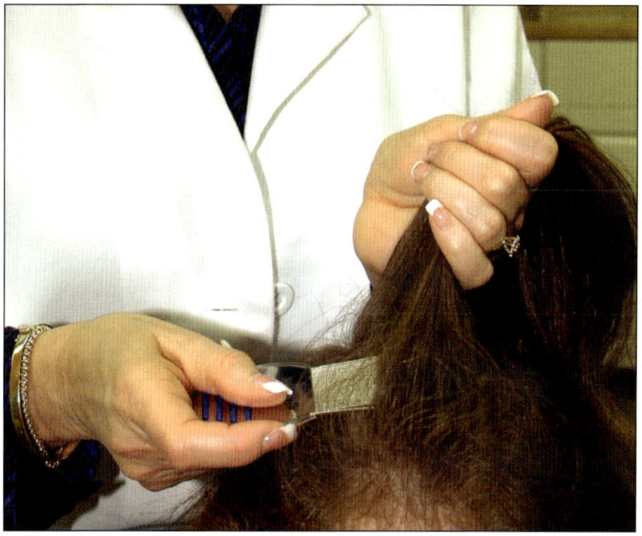

Hold the hair securely away from the scalp and comb from the scalp all the way to the ends.

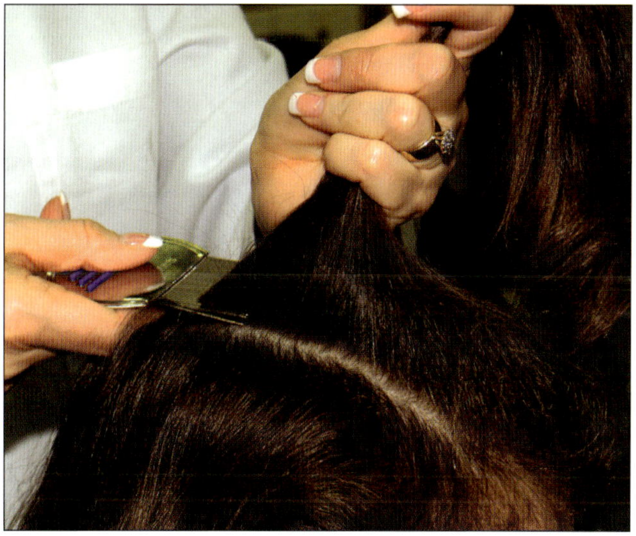

By combing from all angles, around the two inch section, you are able to capture any bugs that sought refuge in this area.

Don't despair—you're almost there! Once you have completed this final examination add one more dose of product and once again comb through thoroughly. In our office we prefer to use a second clean comb for this step. If your product packaging stresses using the entire bottle (and you still have product left over), this would be the time to finish it up. Once again, give the individual you are treating a paper towel. Tell them to cover their eyes and tilt their head back.

Proceed as follows:

Apply an additional dose (or remainder of product if recommended by the manufacturer) of **treatment** product to the hair. If the individual had a severe infestation, particularly if they had a large population of nymphs, a little stronger, but still safe, product could be used. It is not necessary to over-saturate the hair (we prefer not to) as long as the hair is moist enough to comb through easily. Be careful not to allow any product to have contact with skin areas, other than the head. Many products, while safe on the tougher skin of our scalp, will irritate or cause a rash on the softer skin of our neck and back. Use the lice comb and comb against the scalp at a 90-degree angle. Positioning the comb lightly against the scalp, comb in multiple directions—moving in backwards, downwards, and upward motions. During the **comb-out** check the comb often for **evidence** of missed nits or bugs. Your goal is to ensure that once you complete the entire **treatment process** the individual is left with a lice-free environment. If any **evidence** is seen on the comb, continue combing, being careful to always comb ALL the way to the end of the hair. Do so until a **clean comb-out** is achieved. One additional safety net is to comb a total of 20 swipes with no further **evidence.** If anything is found, start the count over. Keep in mind that if the comb is removed prior to reaching the ends of the hair, you are allowing opportunities for bugs to escape!

Pull the individual's hair back into a braid, ponytail, or bun to ensure hair does not get in their eyes. They are now safe to return to their daily activities.

Do's and Don'ts for lice treatment and prevention:

Do:

<u>Wash the product out of the hair prior to going to bed</u> (sooner if directed to by product packaging). We generally leave the product on the hair while the individual drives home. This is fine if you are using a safe, non-toxic product. **WARNING:** If you are treating with a pesticidal product, leave on only as instructed. To leave product on longer than the specified time serves no purpose and could prove harmful for the individual being treated.

<u>Keep the head back when rinsing product out of the hair</u>. While a product may be safe and non-toxic, it is not intended to have contact with the eyes. Products such as enzyme-based ones are irritants. Enzyme in the eyes will feel much like sand.

<u>Get in a good habit of combing</u>. "A comb a day keeps the lice away!" Since you are new at this you might want to take 15 minutes each day for the first three to four days. Beyond that, comb every two to three days for the next three weeks. The life cycle of head lice is three weeks. Combing (and re-checking if you find something) during that time allows you to remove any missed **evidence** prior to it causing a new infestation. Beyond that, keep combing two to five minutes once or twice a week--forever! That way, if your child is ever exposed again, you will identify it early and prevent it from escalating or spreading to others.

<u>Communicate with family and friends</u>. Encourage them to get their hair checked as well, and treat only when necessary. Remind those treated that it's not just about where they got head lice but also who they gave it to as well. One of the many reasons people experience recurrent infestations is because they fail to alert those around them. Since you more than likely received lice in this circle of friends, you most likely shared it there as well and are more likely to get it again. As we like to say, "Head lice is the gift that keeps on giving, so help stop the spread by encouraging your friends to get checked, too!"

Don't:

Let children (especially little girls) sit in the tub while rinsing product out of the hair. Products are tested and intended for limited body absorption. Girls have the added risk of urinary tract infections if they rinse the product out while sitting in a bathtub. Encourage them to wash their hair in the shower or sink. If they must do so in the tub, keep the tub drain open.

Let your guard down too soon. **Follow-up re-checks** are an important part of the **treatment process,** even if you think you did an excellent job. The only way to effectively ensure that no further exposure exists is through **follow-up re-checks**.

OK, so now you ask: What do I do with the bucket of bugs? How much cleaning is necessary? What about my pets? The questions can be endless and therefore we have included them in the question-and-answer section in the back of the book. Don't worry about your pets, keep cleaning to a minimum, and as far as the bucket? In our office we dump it down the toilet. I always joke with the children we treat that one day a giant louse will come out at us! Hey, maybe they'll make a movie about it!

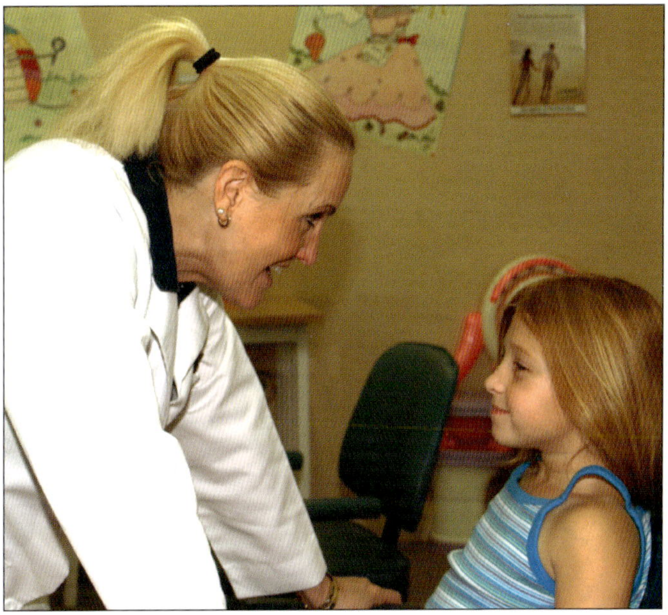

Ms. Shepherd requires that all of her staff strive to better educate the children.

"Lice can happen to anyone! It is not your fault!"

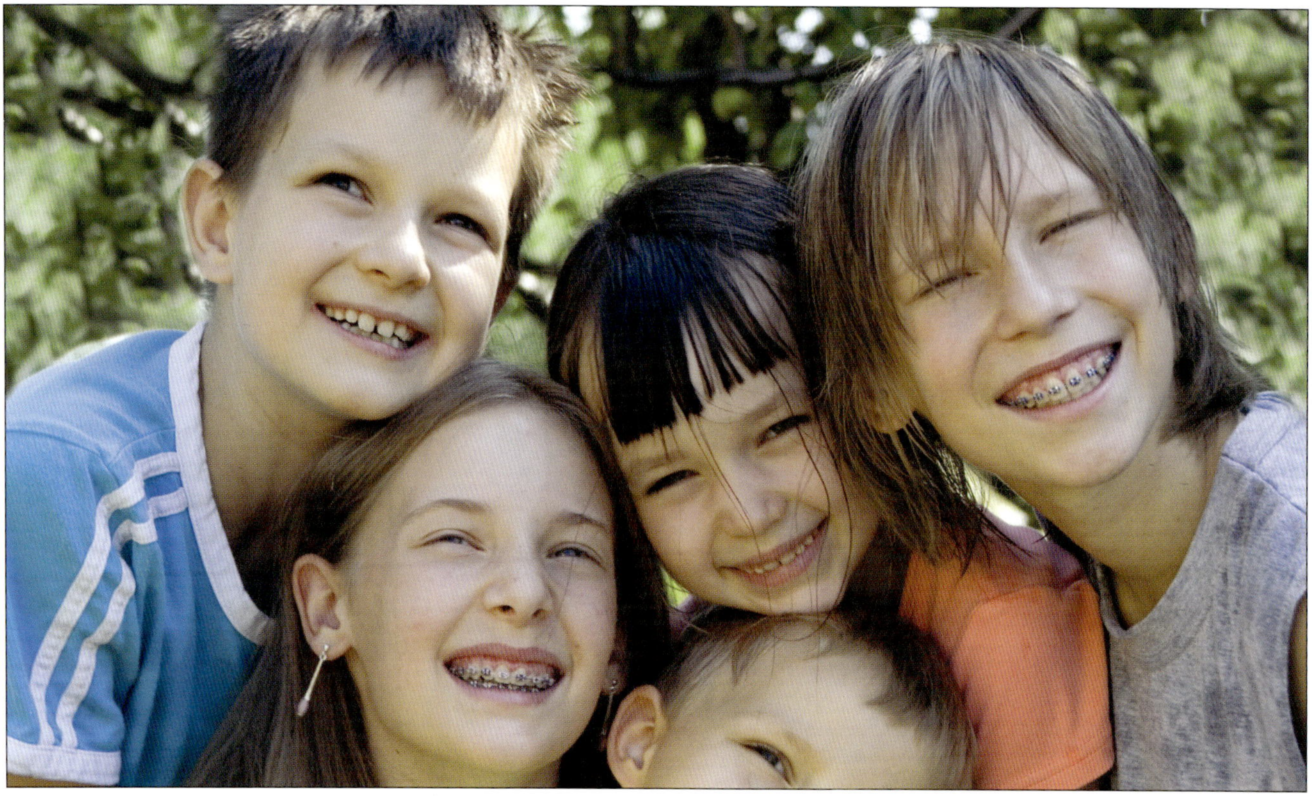

5

FOLLOW-UP RE-CHECK PROCEDURES

For Long Haired Individuals

For short-haired individuals, see procedures on page 83 adapted for that length of hair.

Tools Used: detangler comb, wooden stick, lice comb, non-toxic mint spritz, non-toxic shampoo (if needed), water bucket, and hair tie (not all these tools may be needed). To purchase needed items, check your local pharmacy, beauty supply store or visit: www.licesloutions.org.

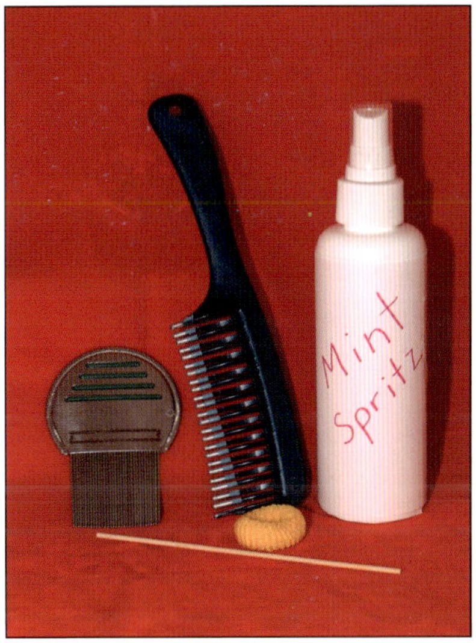

Tools for a follow-up re-check include a quality lice comb, wooden stick, hair tie, detangler comb and mint spritz.

Purpose: A **follow-up re-check** can be performed any time after a **treatment**, but under no circumstances should you allow more than five to seven days to pass after an initial **treatment process** without having done at least one **follow-up re-check**. The purpose of a **re-check** is to ensure that there was nothing left behind and that the individual has not had further contact with other active cases of head lice. The procedure for a **re-check** is very similar to that of a **head check**, with the exception that in a **re-check** the caregiver works with very thin layers of hair and removes any **evidence** if found. Additionally, a **comb-out** is done at the beginning of the **re-check process** to alert you to a potential problem and again at the end to ensure that nothing was missed during your visual examination. Additional product is added only if needed. No further **treatment** is needed if the individual adheres to the required time frame for subsequent **follow-up re-checks**. Depending on the length of the individual's hair, it may be positioned in an imaginary ponytail and re-checked in thin layers (for longer hair) or small sections (for shorter hair).

During the **follow-up re-check process**, the caregiver looks for any **evidence** of head lice. If any bugs are found, the caregiver removes and disposes of them into the water bucket. A **follow-up re-check** generally lasts from 15 to 30 minutes. Keep in mind that if you are able to do this in a timely but efficient manner, there is less chance of wearing yourself out or frustrating the individual being checked.

FOLLOW-UP RE-CHECKS ARE DONE ON DRY HAIR ONLY.

A **follow-up re-check** for long haired individuals consists of the following steps:

Comb the tangles out of the hair with a detangler comb. If the hair is wet, blow-dry it completely first. Nits and bugs are easier to spot on a dry head of hair.

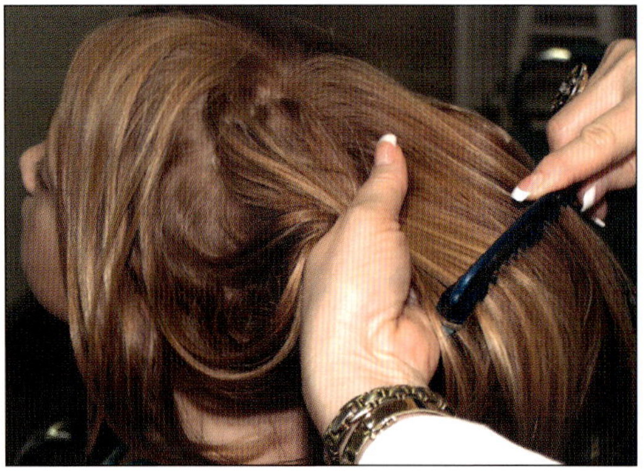

Detangle the hair before starting your **follow-up re-check**.

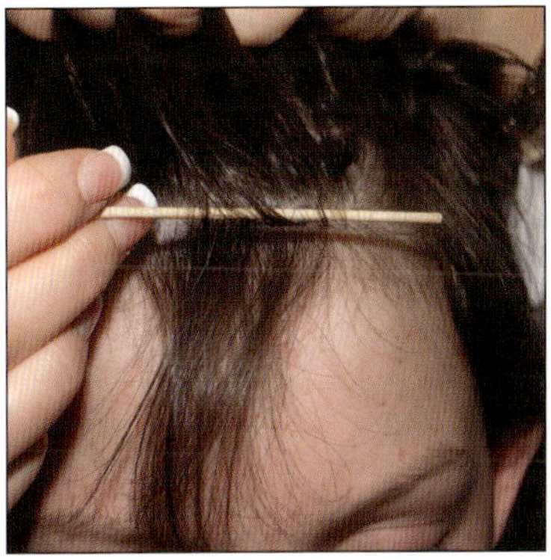 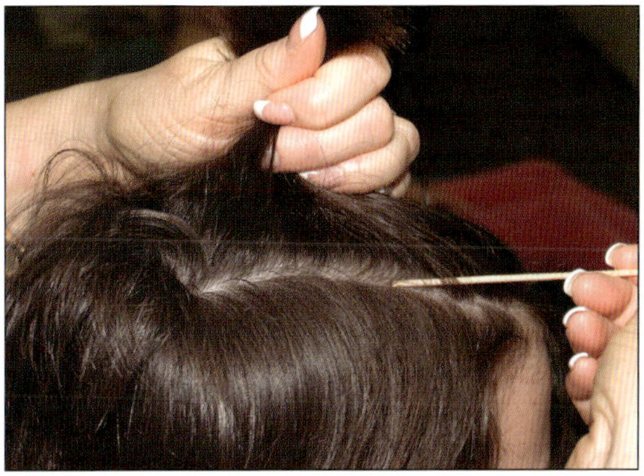 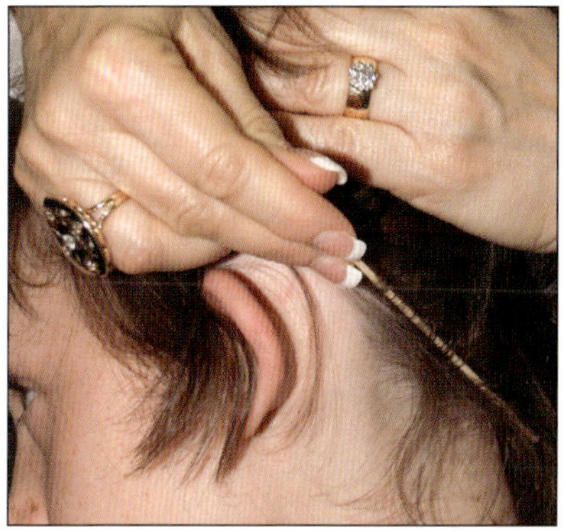

Hot Spots are favorite areas for lice to lay their eggs; left is the bangs, middle is the crown, top right is the ears and right is the nape of the neck.

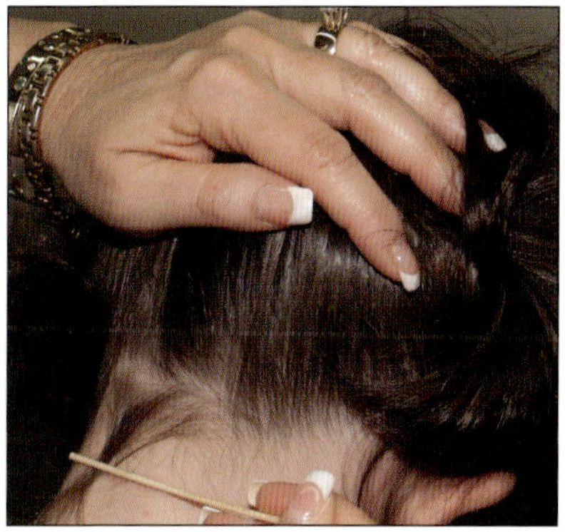

Dry comb the hair with the lice comb for approximately one or two minutes or around 20 strokes as you move around the head of hair. Starting at the bang area, comb back and down to the end of the hair shaft. Comb, look at the comb, comb, look at the comb. Focus on the **hot spots** (favorite areas for lice to congregate and lay their eggs). Comb approximately three swipes in each area: bangs, crown, ears and nape of neck. Doing so quickly alerts you if reinfestation has occurred; thus, a warning sign to you that extra care should be taken. While you need to do a quick comb of the entire head, these areas are the most likely to harbor **evidence**.

As in previous steps, position the teeth of the comb gently against the scalp and comb at a 90-degree angle all the way to the end of the hair. Combing should occur in backward, downward, and upward motions. During this **comb-out process**, check the comb often for **evidence** of head lice. If bugs are found, rinse the comb in the water bucket. Unlike a **head check**, in the **follow-up re-check process** you continue combing out until no more **evidence** is found (this is called a **clean comb-**

out). If no **evidence** is found, the caregiver can set the lice comb aside and proceed with a visual examination.

During the **follow-up re-check process** there is always the possibility of finding **evidence**. If you see nits or bugs, don't panic. (Remember you are doing this in hopes of finding **evidence**--should it exist.) To remove, use your fingernails and grasp the nit, pulling it all the way down the strand of hair and off the head. Be careful to confirm that the nit was removed by checking your finger, keeping in mind that a nit off the hair looks similar to a tiny tadpole. What appears to be a tail is actually the fixative glue that holds the nit in place. When the nit is removed, the glue comes with it, refusing to give up its hold on the nit. Remove bugs with your fingernails or (as was done in the **treatment process**), slide the teeth of the comb under the bug and slowly comb to the end of the strand of hair. Carefully dispose of bugs into the water bucket. If a bug becomes wedged in the comb, place the comb under the water in your water bucket. You can fan the teeth of the comb with your thumb for easier removal of the bug. A little known fact is that bugs tend to fall to the bottom of the bucket while nits settle along the top edge.

Start from the base of neck and work your way up, securing the hair with one hand and positioning it high on the head in an imaginary ponytail. (Since I am right handed, I prefer to grasp the hair with my left hand and pull down thin layers with my right hand. This is a personal choice based on whether you are right- or left-handed, and it doesn't matter which hand you use as long as you achieve the desired end results). The caregiver holds the hair in this manner during the entire **follow-up re-check process.** Using your free hand, pull down thin layers of hair with either a wooden stick, tooth of the lice comb or a fingernail (this is a personal preference). {Reminder: Remove any **evidence** of head lice and dispose of all bugs into the water bucket}.

As you work your way up the head, begin by pulling thin layers of hair from the bottom of the neck area, as well as around the ears and sideburns. Pulling thin layers from side to side allows you to move evenly upward around the head. (While performing **follow-up re-checks**, keep in mind that if bugs still exist, they may move to the top of the head. Therefore, an additional comb-out is done close to the mid-line area, once you reach the top of the head. This process rarely takes less than 15 minutes and can take 30 minutes or more depending on the thickness of the hair.

Understand that if you missed a nit, it has had a week's worth of hair growth, now making the nit more visible to the naked eye. Be sure to talk to the individual while doing this procedure. The process can be stressful, especially if you are finding **evidence** of head lice. Speaking positively to them helps them relax and stay calm. Remind them that this is why **follow-up re-checks** are so important. While there is always the risk that something was missed, there is an even greater risk that they still have contact with someone else who also has head lice. Like a bad cold, it can be handed back and forth. The best way to keep this from happening is to continue to monitor the individual's head of hair.

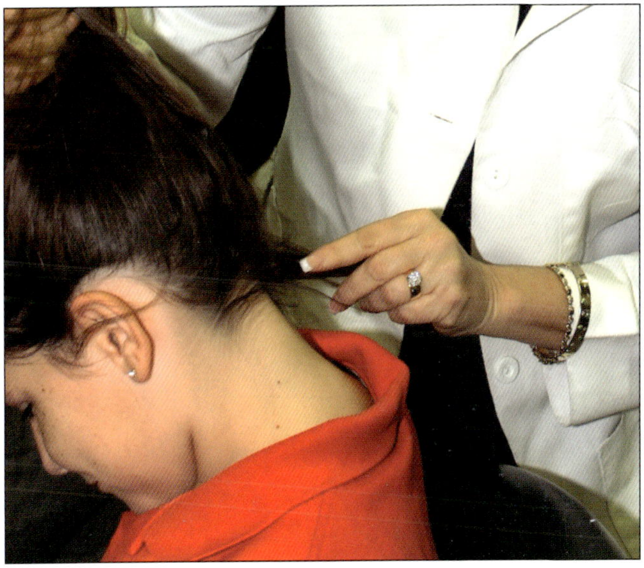

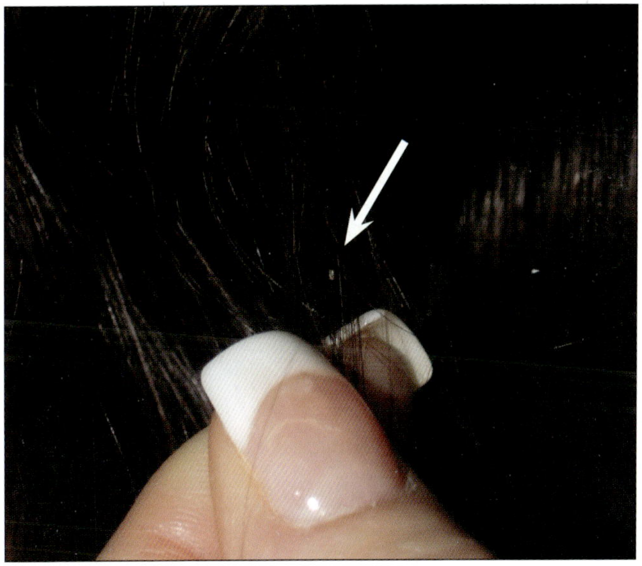

By holding the hair in an imaginary ponytail and working your way towards the top, you are able to find nits that are hidden within the layers of hair.

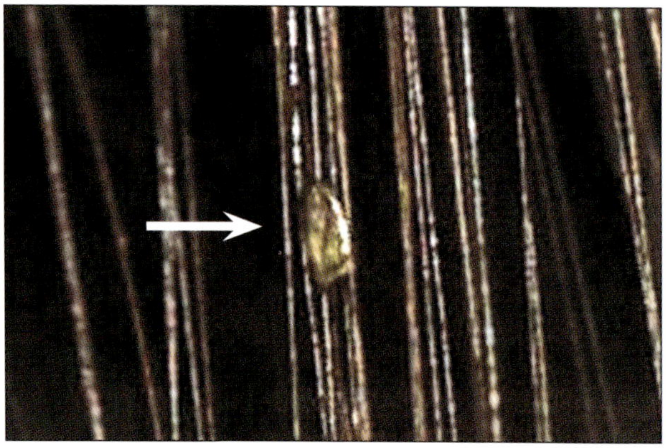

An isolated nit will often indicate a 'missed' nit. Like a needle in a haystack, a nit on dark hair can be extremely difficult to identify.

When doing a **follow-up re-check**, it is worth noting the position of any nits you find. Did you find one here and one there, for example, one or two in the bangs, another at the crown, and maybe one over the right ear? If so, these are considered missed nits. Pull them and move on. If, however, you could place an imaginary quarter over the nit and find three or more nits within the circumference of that space, this indicates a new lay. It also means that you need to be more concerned that an adult louse exists. Be extra careful in your approach to ensure that all bugs are removed. Let the individual know that you are concerned for their wellbeing. Ask if they have experienced any problems, such as finding a bug or excessive itching, and pay close attention to any area in which the individual has expressed concern. Ask them about possible contacts. Who have they been in contact with since you last saw them? This is especially important if third stage or adult bugs are found, as this indicates the likelihood of exposure from another person.

Once you reach approximately one inch from each side of the middle part of the head, take the lice comb and again comb thoroughly throughout that entire area, working your way around the section in a circular motion to ensure the entire section was combed completely. This time, however, instead of combing down and out, as was done in the **final re-check** of your **treatment**, you will comb towards the middle (or part) and then up and out to the ends. Thoroughly combing the area helps ensure that no bugs have made their way to the top of the head. When **comb-out** of this area is complete, finish working your way towards the middle until there is no more hair left to examine.

If the individual has bangs, it is now time to check them. Hold the bangs up with one hand or simply push them back, holding them back as you work your way through this section. Start checking the bangs by pulling thin layers forward until there are no more layers to examine. Remember this is a very common area to find additional nits, so look carefully.

Next is the **final comb-out** of the entire head of hair. Give the individual a paper towel to cover their eyes and ask them to tilt their head back.

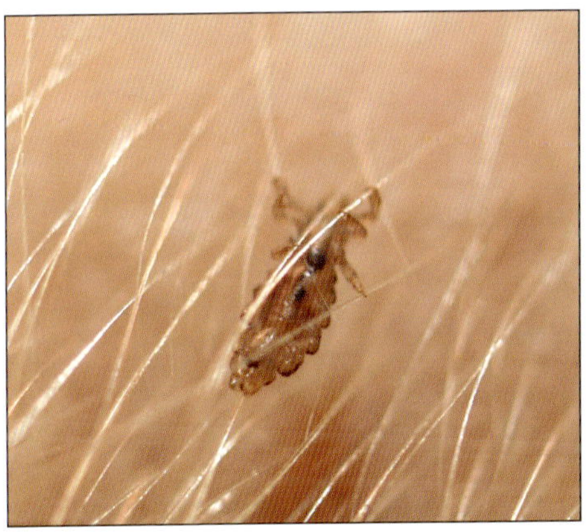

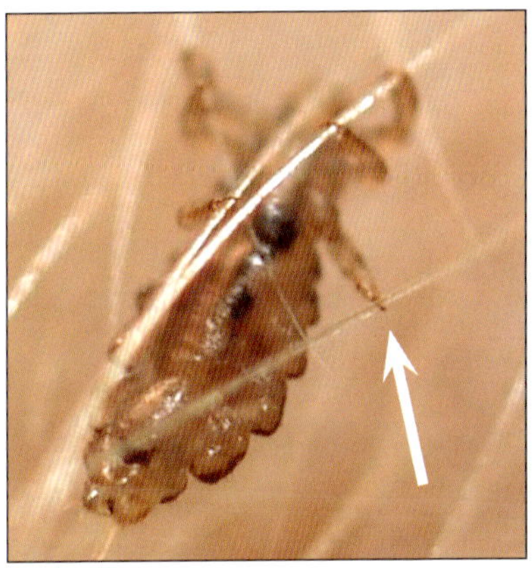

During the **follow up re-checks**, it is not uncommon to find a bug or two on the head. Usually this indicates that there is ongoing contact with other lice-infested individuals.

Left: louse clinging to the hair shaft. Right: enlargement shows the claws of the louse wrapped around the hair

Upon completion choose one of the following comb-out options:

If bugs are not found during the ***follow-up re-check***, lightly spray the hair with a non-toxic mint spritz around the entire head of hair. This will make the **comb-out** easier. It will also send an overlooked bug into motion. Once a bug is moving, it is far easier to **comb out**. If you find a bug during the **comb-out** process, change to the instructions for "bug found."

If bugs are found during the ***follow-up re-check***, apply a non-toxic lice product on the hair until the entire head of hair is dampened (do not over-saturate). It is not necessary to re-treat just because you found a couple of bugs. This merely indicates that exposure to another individual with an active case of head lice still exists - what we call "crossover contamination." A new treatment would be warranted only if the problem were to be neglected, allowing head lice to multiply. Just make sure you have removed everything. Thorough **re-checks** must continue until you have at least two weeks, but preferably three, with no further **evidence** found.

Proceed as follows:

Place the teeth of your lice comb gently against the scalp and comb from the scalp to the end of the hair. Continue to comb the hair in multiple directions - using backward, downward, and upward motions. Doing so ensures that a thorough **comb-out** is achieved. For added safety, comb hair a minimum of 20 swipes without any **evidence** of head lice. If evidence is found, reset the count from the beginning.

When combing the hair, use caution as you place the teeth of the comb gently against the scalp area. Never allow the comb to dig into the scalp of the individual you are treating. It should be a light pass that has contact with the head but does not scrape or damage it.

During the **comb-out process** check the comb often for any **evidence** of head lice. (If bugs are found, remove them and continue combing until no further **evidence** is found.)

Once completed, comb the hair back with a detangler comb and, if possible, put the hair into a ponytail, braid, bun, or similar hairstyle. If using a non-pesticidal product, leave it on the head after The *Shepherd* Method™ treatment process. That way, if a bug was missed it still has direct exposure to the solution on the hair. Equally important and, hopefully more likely, it provides extra protection for the individual, as their head may have contact with contaminated items such as the car seat. I want to emphasize that fewer than 5% of the cases come from such contact. It is a rare possibility. My only concern is to promote measures that err on the side of caution. This is just one more step toward that goal. At Lice Solutions, we recommend that our clients leave the product in the hair for at least two hours. The main reason we do this is to ensure that their hair has added protection when they leave our facility. Since I realize there will be some individuals who use this book as a treatment guide for their own business opportunity, I felt it necessary to point these facts out.

When rinsing out the product, be sure the individual keeps their head tilted back to avoid the risk of the product running into their eyes. Remind them that it is imperative they have their hair **re-checked** in two to three days, and no more than one week, as concern with ongoing contact still exists.

You have now completed the **follow-up re-check process**. Be careful as you move forward not to let your guard down. **Follow-up re-check**s should be done once or twice a week for three consecutive weeks with NO further **evidence** found. Beyond that, comb regularly (preferably two to five minutes once or twice a week) forever. That way if your child is ever exposed again, you will identify it before it has a chance to escalate or spread to others.

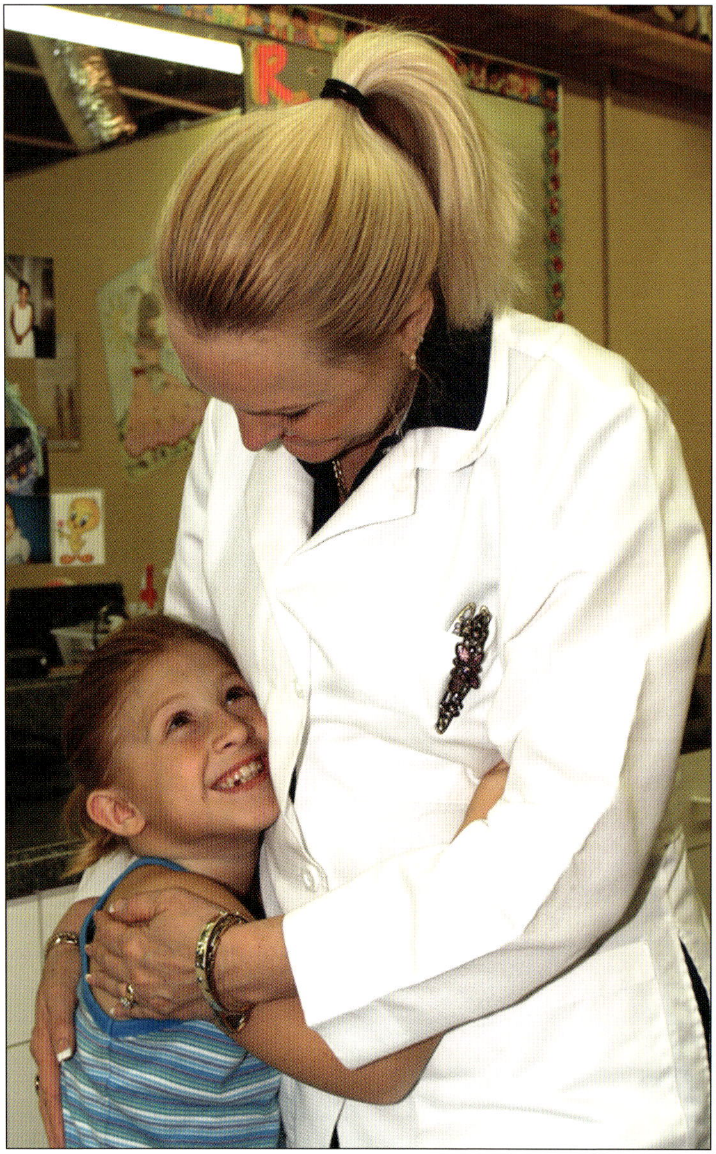

Ms. Katie is always receiving hugs from the children, and she encourages them to hug. Keep safe by tying your hair back avoiding direct hair to hair contact.

FOLLOW-UP RE-CHECK PROCEDURES

Adapted for Short-Haired Individuals

This technique is used when working with hair that is too short to grasp. The procedure for a **follow-up re-check** is very similar to that of a **head check**, with the exception that the caregiver works with thinner layers of hair and removes any **evidence** as they work their way through the hair. Additionally, a **comb-out** is done at the beginning to alert you to a potential problem and again at the end of the **follow-up re-check process** to ensure that nothing was missed during your visual examination. Additional product should be added only if needed. No further **treatment** is needed if the individual adheres to the required time frame of **follow-up re-checks**. Depending on the length of the individual's hair, it may be positioned in an imaginary ponytail within smaller sections, and **re-checked** in thin layers (for slightly longer hair) or small sections (for very short hair).

FOLLOW-UP RE-CHECKS ARE DONE ON DRY HAIR ONLY.

A **follow-up re-check** for short haired individuals consists of the following steps:

Comb any tangles out of the hair with a detangler comb. If their hair is wet, blow-dry it, as nits and bugs are easier to see on a dry head of hair.

Using the lice comb, place the teeth of the comb gently against the scalp and comb throughout the hair. It is important to comb at least two to three swipes in each of the **hot spots** (favorite spots for lice to lay eggs), combing from the scalp, holding the comb at a 90-degree angle. Move the comb in multiple directions--using backward, downward, and upward motions. Comb all the way through to the ends of the hair if any length exists. During the **comb-out,** check the comb often for **evidence** of lice or nits. Comb, look at the comb, comb, look at the comb. Rinse the comb in the water as needed.

If bugs are found, place them immediately in the water bucket. Continue the comb-out until no more **evidence** is found (this is called a **clean comb-out**).

Keep in mind that during the **follow-up re-check process**, there is always the possibility of finding **evidence** of head lice. If you find a nit, use your fingernails to remove it and you can drop it on the floor for later cleanup (there is no need to put them in the water bucket, as they will not re-attach themselves, and doing so slows down the process). If a louse is found, remove it with your nails or lice comb. Carefully dispose of all bugs into the water bucket.

Take your left hand (assuming you are right-handed) and place it on the individual's forehead. Push the hair back off the forehead, holding it down in the process (similar to the bangs technique). Depending on the length of the hair, pull the hair forward in thin layers with either a wooden stick or your fingernail (this is a personal preference). Continue to pull thin layers of hair, while simultaneously moving your hand back towards the crown of the head. Carefully examine the hair and scalp thoroughly as you work your way through the hair. This area is completed when the crown has been reached.

Next check the side areas on the front of the head. Generally, we prefer to check the right side first, although it does not matter which side is done first, as long as both sides are checked thoroughly. Check the sides from the sideburns around the ears, moving upward in the same manner applied in the previous step. Be sure to check from the hairline of the face to the hair lining the ear area. Once you have completed the right side of the head, move to the left side and repeat the process. (If you always work in the same direction, there is never a question as to what has been completed should you get distracted or another individual takes over the **treatment**.)

Move on to check the back of the head. Ask the individual you are checking to tilt their head forward. Place your left hand (assuming you are right-handed) at the back of the neck and push the hair upward. Begin pulling thin layers from one side of the head to the other and carefully move up the middle of the head towards the top of the crown. When the crown is reached, this section is done.

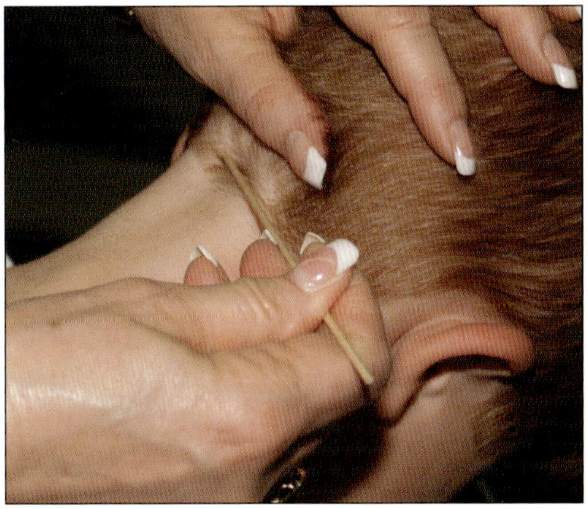

Short hair is no exception, when it comes to finding nits.

Finishing up with the back sides of the head, place one hand on the right side of the back of the head behind the ear area and push the hair in an upward motion while holding the hair firmly. Carefully pull thin layers from the base of the neck and around the ear area, working your way upward toward the crown of the head. When the crown has been reached, this part is done. Continue the same technique for the other side of the head, repeating the process. Keep in mind that head lice prefer to lay eggs on the underside of the hairs. Examining the hair from this direction is absolutely essential.

Your **follow-up re-check** is completed only after the **final comb-out** on the entire head has been satisfactorily achieved. Hand the individual you are treating a paper towel. Have them cover their eyes and ask them to tilt their head back.

Upon completion, choose one of the following comb-out options:

If bugs <u>are not found</u> during ***follow-up re-check***, lightly spray the hair with a non-toxic mint spritz around the entire head of hair. This will make the **comb-out** easier. It will also send an overlooked bug in motion. Once a bug is moving, it is far easier to comb out. If you find a bug during the **comb-out** process, change to the instructions for "bug found."

If bugs <u>are found</u> during ***follow-up re-check,*** apply a non-toxic lice product on the hair until the entire head of hair is dampened (do not over-saturate). It is not necessary to re-treat just because you found a couple of bugs. This would merely indicate exposure to another individual with an active case of head lice. A new treatment would be warranted only if these lice were neglected and allowed to multiply. We refer to this type of exposure as "crossover" contamination. You do, however, want to ensure that you have removed everything. Thorough **re-checks** must continue until you have at least two weeks, preferably three, with no **evidence** found to ensure no further contact with other lice infested individuals exists.

<u>Proceed as follows</u>:

Place the teeth of your lice comb gently against the scalp, combing from the scalp all the way to the end of the hair length. Holding the comb gently against the scalp, comb the hair in multiple directions--using backward, downward, and upward motions. Doing so ensures that a thorough **comb-out** has been done. For added safety, comb hair a minimum of 20 swipes without <u>any</u> **evidence** of head lice. If **evidence** is found, the count should be reset from the beginning.

When combing the hair, be careful to place the teeth gently against the scalp. Never allow the comb to dig into the scalp of the individual you are treating. It should be a light pass that has contact with the head but in no way scrapes or damages the scalp.

During the **comb-out process** check the comb often for **evidence** of head lice. (If you find bugs, remove them and continue combing until no further **evidence** is found.)

Once completed, comb the hair back with a detangler comb and, if possible, put hair into a ponytail, braid, bun, or similar hairstyle. If the product you've used is non-pesticidal, leave it on for two hours after the *Shepherd Method*™ treatment process. That way, if you missed a bug it still has direct exposure to the solution. Equally important, and hopefully more likely, it allows extra protection for the individual, as their head may make contact with contaminated items such as the car seat. I want to emphasize that fewer than 5% of the cases come from such contact. It is a rare possibility. My only concern is to promote measures that err on the side of caution. At Lice Solutions, we recommend our clients leave the product in the hair for at least two hours. The main reason we do this is to ensure that their hair has added protection when they leave our facility. Since I realize there will be some individuals who use this book as a treatment guide for their own business opportunity, I felt it necessary to point these facts out.

When rinsing out the product, be sure the individual keeps their head tilted back to avoid risk of the product running into their eyes. Remind them that it is imperative they have their hair **re-checked** in preferably two to three days, and not more than one week, as concern with ongoing contact still exists.

You have now completed the **follow-up re-check process**. Be careful as you move forward not to let your guard down. **Follow-up re-check**s should be done once or twice a week for three consecutive weeks with NO further **evidence** found. Beyond that, comb regularly (preferably two to five minutes once or twice a week) forever. That way if your child is ever exposed again, you will identify it before it has a chance to escalate or spread to others.

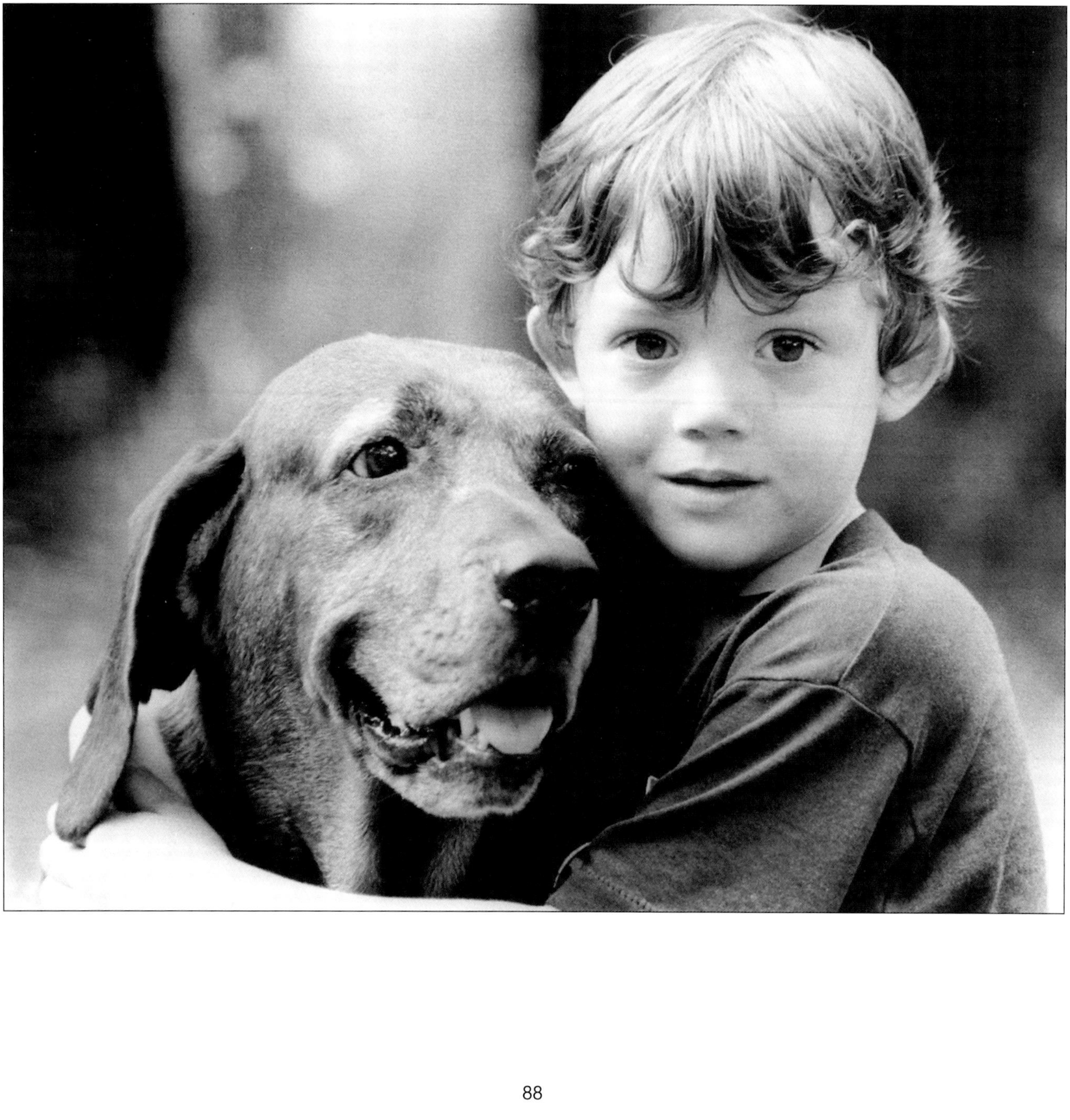

6

The Shepherd Method™ At A Glance

Purpose: To provide you with a quick overview of each phase of the **treatment process** at a glance.

Head Check Procedures

- Detangle hair
- Long hair - grasp in imaginary ponytail
- Short hair - work in sections
- Pull hair down in paper thin layers working towards the top of head
- Examine hair and scalp for any **evidence** of head lice
- With **evidence** - stop **head check** and proceed with **treatment**
- Without **evidence** - comb hair with a good lice comb. Application of mint spritz is recommended.

Treatment process (only after confirmation of head lice)

- Detangle hair
- Protect individual's eyes
- Apply product until hair is damp
- Comb thoroughly until no more **evidence** is combed out
- Section hair

- Cover left side of head
- Work from top to bottom on Section 1
- Comb, feel, shade, flip and clip
- Repeat process Sections 2 through 4, removing all **evidence**
- Remove clips
- Blow hair dry
- **Re-check** similar to **head check**
- Protect individual's eyes
- Apply additional treatment product
- **Final comb-out**
- Tie hair back if possible or wash as normal

Follow-up Re-check Procedures

- Detangle hair
- Comb with good head lice comb - pay attention to **hot spots**
- Check hair per length instructions
- Remove **evidence** if found
- With bugs - apply additional product if necessary
- Without bugs - comb hair with a good lice comb. Application of mint spritz is recommended.

7

"THE SHEPHERD METHOD™"

Definitions

The *Shepherd* Method™: A safe, non-toxic means of treating head lice, **The *Shepherd* Method™** utilizes a **strand-by-strand** combing technique that ensures every hair has been examined and all lice and nits have been removed. **The *Shepherd* Method™** ensures that the hair has been **checked** and **re-checked**, allowing the individual to be treated effectively the first time.

Head Check: The examination of an individual's head for head lice or nits prior to administering any form of lice **treatment**. A positive **head check** indicates the presence of lice or nits and therefore **treatment** is needed. A negative **head check** indicates **NO evidence** was found, therefore **NO treatment** is necessary.

Treatment: The actual process of applying a lice product and combing the hair for the purpose of removing all lice and nits.

Evidence: The findings of nits or bug(s), which indicates the presence of a head lice infestation.

Nit-Picking: The tedious task of painstakingly going through the hair, picking nits one at a time. This technique generally uses one's fingernails to remove nits.

Comb-Out: The act of running a lice comb through one's hair to ensure no lice or nits exist.

Initial Comb-Out: Combing with the lice comb at the beginning of a **treatment process**. This generally takes approximately 15 minutes but can take additional time depending on the length and thickness of the hair. The severity of the infestation also plays a role in time needed to successfully remove the majority of head lice and/or nits.

Final Comb-Out: Combing with the lice comb at the end of a **treatment process** to ensure no nits have been missed and no head lice have escaped the actual **treatment process**. If any **evidence** is found on the comb, the caregiver continues combing until a **"clean" comb-out** is achieved.

Clean Comb-Out or Clean Comb: The point at which the caregiver sees no more nits or bugs on the lice comb during the **Comb-Out** process. Generally this is accomplished when you have 20 clean swipes of the comb with no further **evidence** removed.

Final re-check: A **final re-check** is done immediately after the **treatment** is completed. The purpose is to ensure that no further **evidence** has been left behind. A **final re-check** generally takes 20 to 30 minutes but could take more or less time depending on the thickness of the individual's hair.

Follow-up re-check: Examining hair any time in the days or weeks following a lice **treatment** to ensure all lice and nits were removed and that no further contact with other infested individuals exists.

Hot Spots: Favorite areas for bugs to congregate and lay their eggs. These areas include the bangs, the crown of the head, around the ears (particularly on the back side), and the nape of the neck.

Strand by strand: The process of going through the hair in paper thin layers ensuring that all strands of hair have been examined.

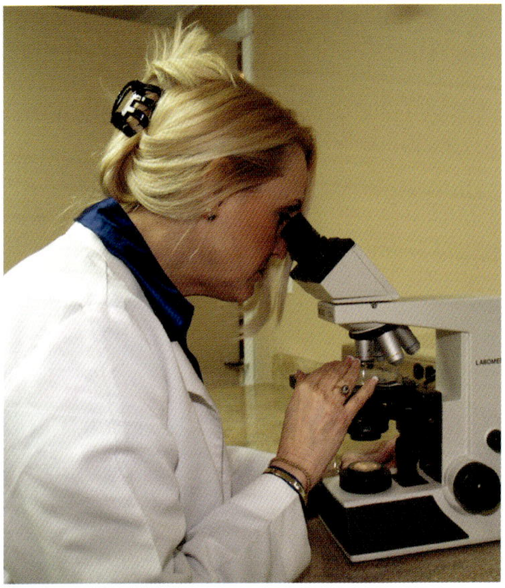

Safer treatment options are a result of ongoing research.

8

QUESTIONS & ANSWERS

1. Head lice are not considered to be life threatening, so why is there so much concern?

Do we really want to live with bugs on our head? Head lice are highly contagious. Whether or not we choose to eliminate them, if we fail to rid ourselves of them we are spreading them to everyone around us. Also, while not generally life-threatening, they can have far-reaching ramifications. Many of those circumstances can lead to other illnesses and yes--in a few situations-- even death.

2. How are head lice spread?

Head lice are primarily spread through head-to-head contact. That is why communicating with individuals with whom you've had recent contact is so important. Fewer than 5% of cases are caused by lice carried on inanimate objects such as brushes, hats, furniture and car seats.

3. How much concern should I have with regard to sharing items like hats or brushes?

Too much emphasis has been placed on sharing items such as hats and brushes. Head lice are primarily spread through head-to-head contact. The bugs can't live off the head for more than 24 hours, and sharing items is not as big an issue as we once thought it was.

4. What, if anything, can people do to help prevent a case of head lice?

You can take many proactive measures. Pulling the hair back is extremely important. It closes a bridge of opportunity that invites lice to spread. Additional measures are (a) obtaining a good lice comb and running it through the hair once or twice a week (b) being aware of the signs of head lice, such as itching, swollen glands, sleepiness after what was assumed to be a good night's rest, a rash at the back of the child's neck (c) being aware of when the child has contact with an active case of head lice, and (d) if a child does have contact, taking extra care in checking them during these time periods.

5. Is there any way to ensure that a person never gets a case of head lice again?

The only way to ensure that you never get it again is to drain all of the blood out of your body! Obviously, that is not an option. As long as you have blood in your body, you are at risk. That's why it is so important to always exercise proactive measures.

6. Can head lice spread disease?

It is believed that head lice do not spread disease. The fact that head lice have a short life span, limited transmission and are host-specific certainly reduces the odds of spreading disease. Some researchers in the field, however, do believe that they can carry diseases, and studies are currently being done in that area to prove this one way or the other.

7. What exactly is a "No Nit Policy" and why does Lice Solutions feel that it is so important?

A "No Nit Policy" means any child with nits is excluded from school. While Lice Solutions supports the "No Nit Policy," we also believe that it needs some modifications, as under current guidelines having just one nit causes the child to have to stay home. We believe that when the nurses have searched thoroughly and found one or two nits, they should pull the nits out and allow the children to return to class. Then the nurse should **re-check** the child at least every three to four days for the next three weeks to ensure that no further contact with other active cases of head lice exists and that the child is truly past it.

8. A lot of states are changing to a live-bug-only policy. What does that mean, and what is Lice Solutions' opinion regarding it?

It is true that many states are changing to a live-bug-only policy. We are not in favor of it, as it is a very dangerous policy. A live-bug-only policy means that whether the child has a nit or not, the child can go to class as long as no one sees a bug on the child's head. The problem is that the bugs are like chameleons; they blend with their environment. You could be looking right at a bug and not see it; they are just too easy to overlook. Children have been sent to our office by the school nurse who swear the child had nits but no bugs. Then we treat them and comb-out 20, 40, even 60 bugs or more.

9. How do parents know if their child has head lice?

Parents should watch for symptoms such as itching, swollen glands, sleepiness after what was assumed to be a good night's rest, or a rash at the back of the child's neck. They should check the head on a regular basis, run a lice comb through the hair once or twice a week, and not let their guard down.

10. What should parents do if they find head lice?

Treat the child as quickly as possible. In doing so you reduce the chance that the lice will spread to others. They should also check other family members to rule them out. They need to communicate with the school nurse, their relatives, neighbors, and the child's closest friends. Keep in mind it's not just where you got head lice, but "whom you gave it to as well." We like to say that it's the gift that keeps on giving. While not the gift any of us want, it is shared nonetheless. Only by taking precautionary measures can we deter it and keep it from endlessly recurring.

11. Who is at risk of getting a case of head lice?

No one is immune from head lice. It's a contact issue. If you have contact with an infested person, you can get it. We have found head lice on people as young as two months and as old as 98 years.

12. Does having head lice mean the individual lives in a dirty home or has poor hygiene?

Absolutely not! A case of head lice arises from contact and has nothing to do with the cleanliness of either one's house or one's person. If anything, it's just the opposite. It is much easier for lice to maneuver on a clean head of hair. Therefore, they prefer this environment. That, however, is not a reason to avoid washing your hair.

Our most severe cases are often found on individuals with poor hygiene. Why? Because they are not disturbing the environment nor are they dealing with the problem. A neglected head of hair is the perfect environment for head lice. Only when it becomes crowded do they look to move to a better environment. As far as the house goes, since head lice do not live off the head, whether your home is clean or dirty makes no difference to them.

13. Can head lice jump or fly?

No, it's another myth associated with head lice. It's anatomically impossible for head lice to jump or fly, as they have no hind legs or wings.

14. When head lice transfer from one head to another, how soon can they start laying eggs?

If the head lice are fertilized females, they can and will begin laying eggs immediately. Another point to keep in mind is that head lice generally travel in harems, often consisting of seven or eight females and one male. With this many egg-laying females laying eight to ten eggs daily, you can see how what starts as a simple case of head lice can escalate very quickly.

15. How do I know if an egg (or nit, as it is commonly called) is viable?

The only way to be certain if a nit is viable is to look at the egg under a microscope. This is one of the main reasons why no-nit policies exist. Obviously, you're not going to stop and examine every nit. So as policy goes, if you see a nit, pull it!

16. If my child gets head lice, can I just shave his/her head?

I don't encourage anyone to shave heads. While some boys might consider that a great option, do we really want to do that to the girls? Even with today's "skater look," many boys would be devastated to give up their locks of hair. Keep in mind that shaving to rid head lice does not mean the hair is cut short—it means it's shaved bald.

17. How many eggs can a head louse lay in a day?

A single female louse lays eggs twice a day, four to five eggs each time. Multiply that by the 10, 20, even 40 or 60 bugs that might be on the head and it's easy to realize how a severe infestation can develop so quickly.

18. How long do head lice live?

A louse, on the head, can live up to 30 days.

19. Where do head lice come from?

Nobody knows for sure where head lice originated. They have been around since the beginning of mankind. Scientists have even found nits on the hair of Egyptian mummies.

20. How can I get my child's school more involved in this health issue?

Talk to your child's school and the school's nurse. Address your concerns and let them know that fighting head lice matters to you. Do this in a calm, rather than an accusing, manner. Remain positive and most importantly, work together! Be careful to stress that your goal is <u>not</u> to place blame but rather to work with them to help develop more proactive measures in hopes of ensuring that <u>ALL</u> children will have a lice-free environment.

Finally, be willing to step up to the plate and assist where help is needed, whether it's checking children's heads, educating families or helping raise funds to ensure all children have the necessary tools and resources to fight head lice. You must be willing to do your part if you truly want to make a difference.

21. If my child has head lice, should I tell the school nurse?

Absolutely tell the school nurse! If you fail to tell the nurse, she won't be aware of it, which means she can't help you by identifying other active cases of head lice. Keep in mind that it's not just about where you got head lice but who you gave it to as well. Unless you're willing to communicate with others that you had head lice, you are at risk of getting it again and again.

22. I've heard the worst part of having head lice is all the cleaning. Is this true?

No. While a good spring cleaning gives you a clean house, it does little to eliminate the head lice problem. The parent's time is better spent on the child's head and communicating with the child's closest friends.

Head lice do not live off the head nor are eggs lying in wait for the perfect moment to hatch and re-infest your family. Lice do not leave your head by choice, and they can't survive for more than 24 hours off the head. They need blood to survive. Likewise a nit, once separated from the head, will die. It needs the warmth of the body to incubate, much like a chicken sitting on an egg.

23. What about products? Is there one that will get everything out?

Wouldn't that be a perfect world? Unfortunately, there is no miracle product. The product merely assists you in your **treatment process**. Therefore, we encourage you to exercise caution and to use safe, non-toxic products when looking at treatment options.

24. What types of products should I look for when shopping?

First and foremost, get a good lice comb. Second, look for safe, non-toxic products. Many non-toxic products are as effective as the toxic ones, including some homeopathic methods. Lice products are not intended as cure-alls but rather as a means of minimizing the tedious task of nit removal. It's worth noting that newer and safer treatment options are entering the market all the time, so keep informed on better alternatives. Beyond that, whatever you do, always exercise caution, and keep it safe!

25. We've already used the common products found in our local pharmacy and they didn't work. Why is that?

Many products currently available have been on the market for as long as 30 years. Partly due to overuse of these products, the bugs have built up a resistance to them. While several products are currently in the developmental stages, bringing an FDA approved product to market is both time-consuming and costly. Until then we must look for safer and more effective alternatives.

26. What can you tell us about home remedies?

There are many home remedies, most of which we don't endorse. Most are messy, time-consuming and no more effective than the safe commercial products available in stores, and in some cases they are just as dangerous, if not more so, than the pesticidal products on the market. If I had to choose one, it would be olive oil; but again, I generally don't encourage using it. There is just no shortcut to eliminating a case of head lice.

27. What is the quickest way to get past a case of head lice?

The term "quick" is not in the head lice dictionary. The best way to get past it as quickly as possible is to treat right the first time and not let your guard down when it comes to **follow-up re-checks**. Tedious, time-consuming nitpicking and checking everyone with whom the person has had contact is the first step toward eliminating head lice. Rushing through a **treatment process** (as the saying goes—haste makes waste), or failing to follow up, guarantees that you will be treating your child again and again. A good comb (when used properly) can eliminate up to 85% of the problem. Even when you think you have done the job right, don't stop checking. The life cycle of lice is three weeks, so keep checking during that time frame.

28. Is it true that itching is the first sign of head lice?

While itching is the most obvious and often the first sign of head lice, it is not always so. Itching is caused by an allergic reaction to the saliva that lice secrete when feeding. Lice saliva keeps the blood meal from clotting, making the feeding process easier. It takes approximately two weeks for enough saliva to build up to cause itching, if one is going to itch. The fact is that as much as 50% of the population never itches with head lice.

29. Whom should I notify if my child has lice?

Notify anyone who has had contact with the child in at least the last two weeks, and preferably during the past month. Beyond that, notify the school nurse, daycare director, camp counselor or any other individual who can assist you in communicating with and checking those with whom your child has been in contact.

30. Does health insurance pay for nit removal services?

At this time, most health insurance companies don't pay for these services. It is still a new procedure, and most companies require a procedure code to process it. That said, most health savings accounts will reimburse the client after services are rendered and receipts submitted. Also, if a physician issues a prescription for nit removal services, some insurance companies will pay for the child's **treatment**. It's certainly worth a try. Finally, if you have enough medical expense to deduct on your taxes, this could be included there, and if you have a court-ordered shared medical with the child's other parent, it is also recognized by the courts as a medical expense.

31. How long can a person have a case of head lice before realizing it?

It is possible to have head lice for years without knowing it, especially if the person does not experience itching. Generally, however, by the time someone identifies head lice, he/she has had head lice for four to eight weeks.

32. Does a case of head lice ever go away by itself?

On rare occasions a case of head lice can go away by itself. More often, however, the case continues to multiply and spread to others.

33. Besides itching, what are some other symptoms of head lice?

Some other symptoms of head lice are low-grade fever, bags under the eyes, swollen glands, a rash at the nape of the neck and falling asleep after a seemingly good night's rest. Head lice are nocturnal, meaning that they are more active at night than during the day. Thus, we toss and turn and in effect do not have a restful night, therefore the saying, "a lousy night's sleep."

34. How much cleaning is necessary when my child has head lice?

Think of your life in a 24-hour window and concentrate only on items that had direct contact with your child during the 24 hours prior to treating them.

As an example: The child was in bed, so you change or wash the sheets. The child took a bath, so you replace the towel. The child brushed his/her hair, so you clean or replace the hairbrush. Also, if your child sleeps with a stuffed animal or a blanket, throw those into a dryer for 30 minutes. As far as carpets and upholstered furniture, just run a quick vacuum or lint remover over them; or place an old sheet over your child's favorite chair or seat. Any of these choices will reduce housework while keeping your home safe.

35. My friend told me she used mayonnaise to get rid of their head lice. What is your opinion of that process?

Mayonnaise is a safe but messy alternative for treating head lice. My opinion: "Do you really want to turn your child's hair into a salad?" There are a lot of equally safe, yet far more effective, options available.

36. Is it true that Afro-American children can't get head lice?

Absolutely not! While it is true that they are less likely to get head lice due to their oval-shaped hair, they are far from immune. Anyone can get head lice. In our office, we see an average of six to eight cases of head lice on Afro-American children each week.

37. Is there a head lice season? If so, when?

While it may seem that we see more cases of head lice during the school months, it is not due to a lice season. Lice happen all year round. However, since children have more contact with each other in a classroom environment than they do during the summer months, we see an increase in numbers during school months. Additionally, there are many schools that still enforce head lice policies, therefore making those numbers more obvious.

38. I've heard that using hairspray prevents head lice. Is that true?

Although hairspray is often thought to be a preventative, it is not. Many people believe that a dirty head of hair can't get head lice and thus they over-apply hairspray, gels and similar products, all of which is a throwback to the myth that Afro-American children can't get head lice. The most you can hope for is that it will keep the hair closer to the scalp, making it less likely to have contact with another. If you must use hairspray, do so in moderation.

39. Do head lice prefer clean hair or dirty hair?

We always ask our clients, "Which is easier to walk on--a clean floor or a dirty, greasy floor?" It's the same with head lice. It's much easier for them to move around on a clean head of hair. This doesn't mean that an individual with a dirty head of hair won't get lice and is certainly no reason to encourage poor hygiene in our children. Head lice need blood to survive. As long as we have blood, we are at risk.

40. Are head lice more prevalent in warmer climates?

The only difference that a warmer climate makes is that the bugs have the ability to move more freely about the hair and therefore can lay eggs throughout the hair. In colder climates they generally stay closer to the scalp. Head lice exist virtually everywhere!

41. Why is it that some people seem to get head lice over and over again while others never do?

There are many reasons why some people seem to get lice repeatedly. First and foremost is the likelihood that they were never past it in the first place. Secondly is the fact that they are likely back in the same environment, sharing close contact with the same individuals, thus exposing themselves to the risk of re-infestation. Additionally, when the bugs feed on us, they leave a scent behind, which attracts other head lice. A good example would be to consider a dog using a fire hydrant. A scent is left that is noticable only to dogs. When the second dog comes along he knows the first dog was there. In the case of head lice no one knows for certain how long the scent lasts. We encourage our clients to be extremely cautious for a period of three weeks and extra careful for 90 days after battling a case of head lice. Finally, bugs must feed on blood. "What type?" you ask. The answer is simple: whatever type they are used to feeding on. Think of a blood transfusion. If you were to receive blood, you must get a blood type that is compatible with yours. To do otherwise could kill you. The same holds true with head lice.

Studies conducted by Terry Meinking found that head lice intentionally avoided an incompatible blood type (especially where the Rh factor is concerned) unless they were starving. Only then did they dare to feed and in doing so assured their sudden death. What Professor Meinking found is that feeding on an incompatible blood type caused their intestinal tracts to explode. Keep in mind, however, that the bug may lay a few nits prior to feeding, and when those nits hatch, they will feed on the new blood type, thus allowing change to take place. Since blood type plays such an active role, it is easy to see how an individual with a common blood type would be more likely to have contact with others who have head lice and share the same blood type. On the other hand, an individual who has a rarer type of blood would be less likely to have contact with others having both head lice and their type of blood.

42. What treatment options are available for my family?

Many **treatment** options are available, including prescription, over-the-counter and homeopathic ones. **Treatment** options include prescription products such as Qwell and Ovide, pyrethrin products like Nix, or permethrin products like Rid, which are available over the counter, as well as a wealth of other safe, non-toxic products including Nit-Free, X-Pel, Lice Free and Lice Cure. Homeopathic methods like olive oil and mayonnaise are popular in many households, but we urge caution when trying home remedies.

We encourage people to use safe, non-toxic products whenever possible. If, however, you could use one tool or product only, we would recommend a good lice comb. The most important thing is that you do something. Head lice left unattended will only escalate and spread to others.

There is no perfect product. The real secret is, know what you are looking for and take the time to treat correctly. We also encourage you to pay close attention to newer and safer alternatives frequently entering the market.

Finally, **never** resort to dangerous **treatments** of the past like kerosene, flea shampoos or insect sprays. Always act wisely and safely!

43. There's been news about a new treatment option called Cetaphil. Does it work?

Cetaphil is a facial cleanser that has received a great deal of attention in the **treatment** of head lice. We have several concerns with this method; first and foremost, it was devised as a scam. Dr. Dale Pearlman, a dermatologist from Menlo Park, California applied a mysterious product (later identified as Cetaphil) to the heads of test subjects and then "shrink-wrapped their hair in it" to suffocate the bugs. Charging his clients a fee to participate in the study, he later admitted that he lied to his peers in hopes of "getting rich quick." While the product did have some impact on adult bugs, it did little if anything to rid people of nits or newly-hatched nymphs. It was no more effective than any other product on the market, since it required multiple and successive **treatments** to provide anticipated results. Finally, we have seen more than a few families that have tried this route only to continue to battle lice weeks, even months later.

44. Is it true that nits closest to the scalp are alive while those away from the scalp are not?

Most likely "yes" but not always. While it is more likely to find nits closer to the scalp, it is not to say that you won't find them an inch or two down the hair shaft, especially in warmer climates where bugs move more freely throughout the hair. Additionally, we can change the position of our hair, ultimately bringing lower hairs to the head lice, as would be the case when we wear our hair in a bun or sleep with it loose around our face. All the bugs know is that it's hair, not where they belong on the strand. We have examined samples of hair with multiple eggs on it only to discover that that the eggs nearest the root were empty, while eggs farther from the scalp were viable. While presenting before the Florida Department of Education, Dr. Shirley Gordon and I were able to demonstrate that the nits farthest from the scalp were not only viable, but under the microscope could be seen breathing!

45. If my child has head lice, should I treat everyone (in the family)?

Don't treat needlessly! We like to ask, "If one family member has a cold, would you give medicine to everyone?" Of course not! What you would do, however, is exercise precautionary measures. The same holds true with lice. Be aware, check, comb, watch for signs, and only if necessary, treat. Do a **head check** first, and only if **evidence** of head lice is identified on that person do we recommend a **treatment**.

46. I treated my daughter using an over-the-counter product and spent many hours combing through her very long hair. It seemed she had a light case, and I did the second treatment ten days later. Yesterday after about a week, I checked her head again and found a few more eggs, repeated the treatment process and washed all linens, etc. What I need to know is, if I find more nits, should I re-treat her again?

You should not continue to re-treat her with the product you used but instead keep looking and combing. The fact that you found more nits does not necessarily mean that she has a new case. It could be nothing more than missed nits. The question is not that you are finding them but how you are finding them. When a louse lays eggs, it lays them in clusters of three to five nits at a time. Imagine taking a quarter and setting it over the nit. If you find additional nits within that area it would be considered a cluster. If you find them in a cluster, comb more and look harder in the quest for the responsible louse. If, however, you find them scattered (for example, one behind the right ear, one in the bangs and one at the nape of neck), then more likely these nits were missed. With a little time for hair growth, a nit that was originally at the root of the hair has now moved far enough away from the scalp to become visible.

The best thing you can do is keep looking and combing every two to three days for the next couple of weeks. If you find a nit, pull it and keep checking. Get a good comb and use it regularly. Incorporate combing into your regular routine and spend two to five minutes (with hair wet) combing once or twice a week, forever!

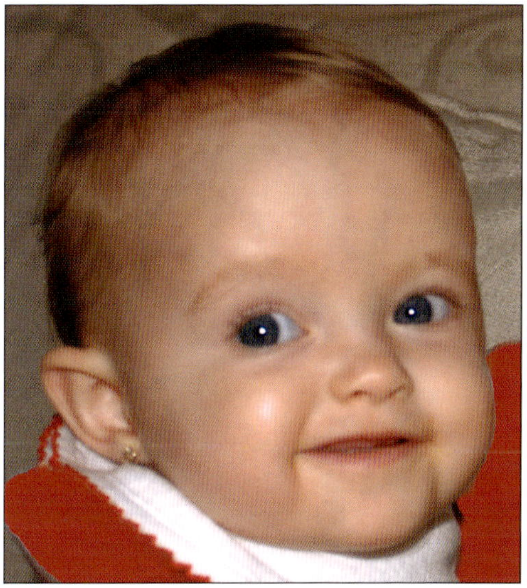

Wishing you a lice-free future!

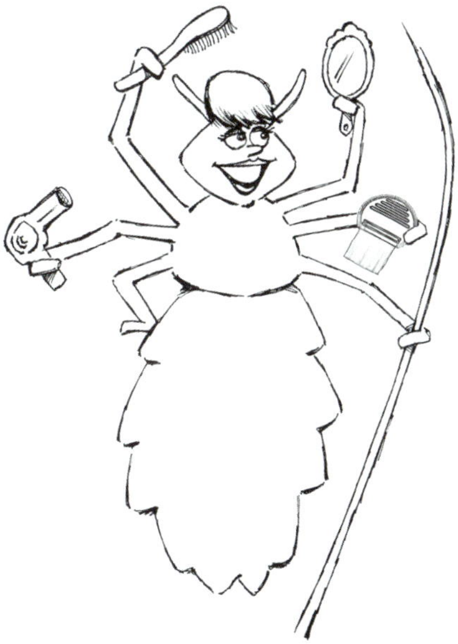

"Remember,
your new best
friend should be a
good lice comb"

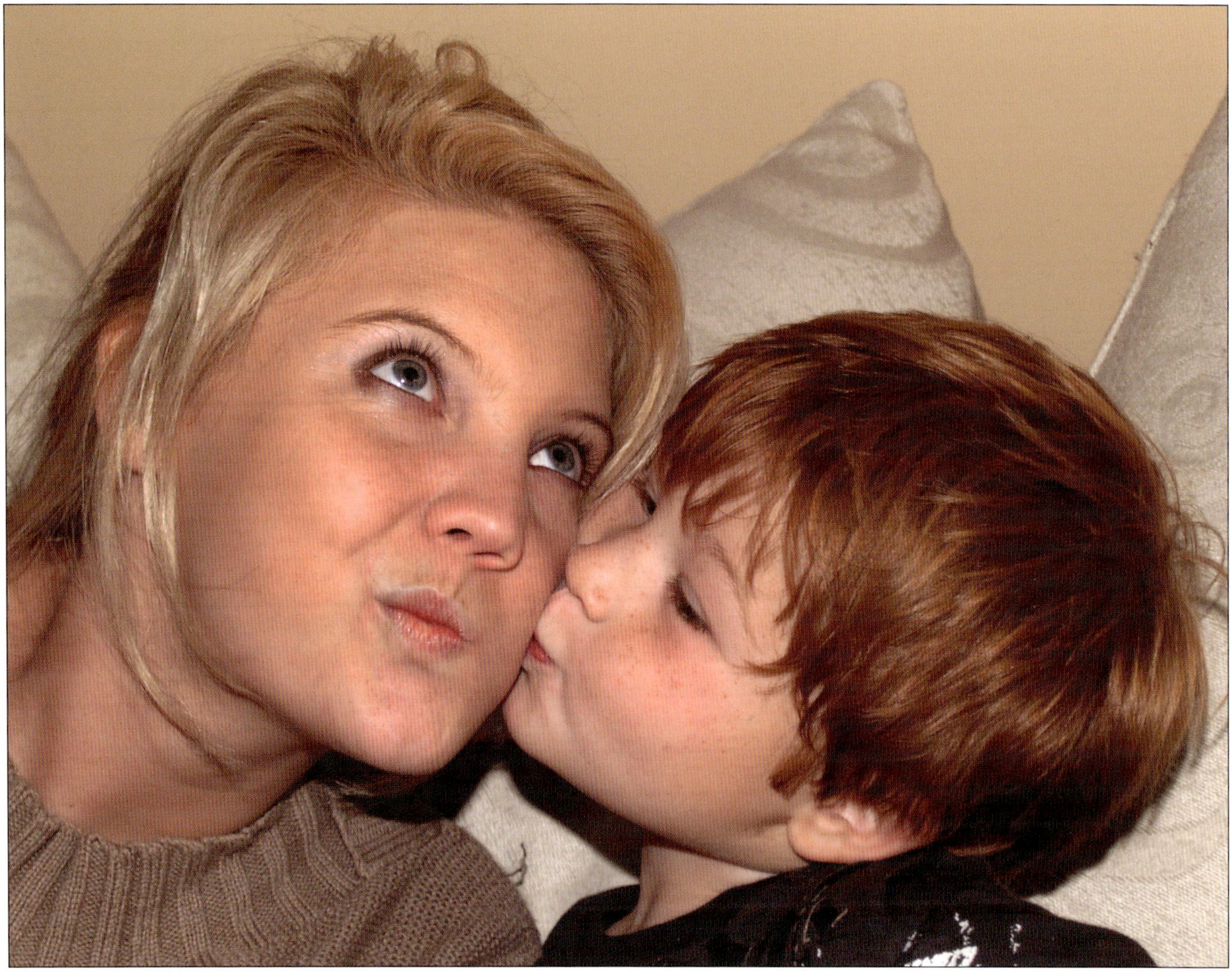

REFERENCES

Although this book was not written as, nor meant to be, a scientific work, many researchers, studies and organizations are referenced within these pages. I would like to give credit to the dedicated scientists who work with lice and to provide additional resources for those persons who need to know more. Hopefully it will help quench the thirst for more in-depth head lice knowledge.

Associated Press. "Lice Lotion Just Snake Oil Scam." Wcco.com 5 Dec. 2005. CBS Broadcasting Inc. 26 Dec. 2008 <http://wcco.com/watercooler/Health/Lice.Dr.2.260683.html>.

Burgess, Ian. "Listing of Publications." BiomedExperts: Scientific Social Networking. 26 Dec. 2008 <http://www.biomedexperts.com/start/PersonDetailpage.aspx?pid=1685603>.

Clark, John M. "Listing of Publications." University of Massachusetts. 23 Dec. 2008 <http://www.bio.umass.edu/mcb/faculty/Clark.html>.

Clayton, Dale H. "Listing of Publications." The University of Utah. 23 Dec. 2008 <http://darwin.biology.utah.edu/PubsHTML/PubsListing.html>.

Cone, Marla. "EPA Bans Lindane for Use as Pesticide." Los Angeles Times [California] 2 Aug. 2006: A16. 26 Dec. 2008 <http://articles.latimes.com/2006/aug/02/nation/na-lindane2>.

Davis JR, Brownson RC, Garcia R, Bentz BJ, and Turner A. "Family pesticide use and childhood brain cancer." Archives of Environmental Contamination and Toxicology 22(3) (APR 1992): 260-66. Abstract. PubMed: MEDLINE PMID: 1616309.

Frankowski, Barbara L. Guidelines for the Prevention and Treatment of Head Lice Infestations. Rep. Sept. 2004. American Academy of Pediatrics. 26 Dec. 2008 <http://www.ajmc.com/files/articlefiles/A78_04FrankowskiS269_S272.pdf>.

Goates, Brad M., Joseph S. Atkin, Kevin G. Wilding, Kurt G. Burch, Michael R. Cottam, Sarah E. Bush, and Dale H. Clayton. "An Effective Nonchemical Treatment for Head Lice: A Lot of Hot Air." Pediatrics 118 (NOV 2006): 1962-970.

Gordon, Shirley C. "Factors contributing to the overuse of chemical pesticides in children with persistent head lice." The Journal of School Nursing 15(5) (DEC 1999): 6-10. Abstract. PubMed: MEDLINE PMID: 10889684.

Gordon, Shirley C. "Shared vulnerability: a theory of caring for children with persistent head lice." The Journal of School Nursing 23(5) (OCT 2007): 283-92. Abstract. PubMed: MEDLINE PMID: 17894526.

"Head-Lice 'Huckster' Draws Criticism for Misleading Behavior", Las Vegas, NV., Daily News Central: Health News, 5, Dec 2005. <http://health.dailynewscentral.com/content/view/0001985/40>.

"Head Lice Shampoo Linked To Leukemia." Consumeraffairs.com/news 17 Jan. 2006. Consumeraffairs.com. 26 Dec. 2008 <http://www.consumeraffairs.com/news04/2006/01/head_lice.html>.

Heavin, Janese. "Lice send 50 home from North Callaway High School." Columbia Daily Tribune [Missouri] 9 Nov. 2006. Columbiatribune.com. 26 Dec. 2008 <http://www.columbiatribune.com/2006/NOV/20061109News001.asp>.

Hoffer, Debbie. "Medical Breakthrough Wipes Out Head Lice, the LouseBuster." Childnparent.com. Child n' Parent. 26 Dec. 2008 <http://www.childnparent.com/read_about/Child+Health/lousebuster>.

Hutchins, Chris. "Healthy Lice Prefer Healthy Kids, Clean Hair." The Palm Beach Post [Florida] 19 Feb. 2002: 5D. Article with expert, Terri Meinking.

Illes, Judith. "A Modern Problem as Old as the Pyramids." Tour Egypt. Association of Egyptian Travel Businesses on the Internet. 23 Dec. 2008.

"Lice: Head Lice: Fact Sheet - CDC DPD." Centers for Disease Control and Prevention. 26 Dec. 2008 <http://www.cdc.gov/lice/head/factsheet.html>.

Meinking, Terri L. "Listing of Publications." Global Health Associates of Miami, Inc. 23 Dec. 2008 <http://www.ghamiami.com/publications.html>.

Mumcuoglu KY, Barker SC, Burgess IE, Combescot-Lang C, Dalgleish RC, Miller J, Roberts RJ, and Taylan-Ozkan A. "International guidelines for effective control of head louse infestations." Journal of Drugs in Dermatology. 6(4) (APR 2007): 409-14. Abstract. PubMed: MEDLINE PMID: 17668538.

Newman, Dan. "School closes due to high number of head lice cases | independent.gmnews.com | Independent." Independent.gmnews.com | Independent | Front Page. 11 Oct. 2006. Independent. 23 Dec. 2008 <http://independent.gmnews.com/news/2006/1011/schools/007.html>.

"The No Nit Policy." Headlice.Org. National Pediculosis Association, Inc. 23 Dec. 2008 <www. headlice.org>.

Reed, David L. "Listing of Publications." Florida Museum of Natural History. 26 Dec. 2008 <http://www.flmnh.ufl.edu/mammals/Publications.html>.

Shepherd, Katie. Comparison Comb Study of the Three Leading Combs Currently on the US Market. Rep. no. GNP2007-01. Aug. 2007. Ginesis Natural Products. 22 Dec. 2008 <http://www.ginesis.com>

Thatcher, Betsy, and Lori Holly. "Two Falls schools report head lice outbreak 63 children and staffmembers are affected." HighBeam Research. 19 Feb. 1999. The Milwaukee Journal Sentinel. 23 Dec. 2008.

USA. Federal Drug Administration. Center for Drug Evaluation and Research. EPA and CDER/FDA Approaches to Acceptable Exposure to Lindane. 16 July 2002. Federal Drug Administration. 23 Dec. 2008 <http://www.fda.gov/cder/drug/infopage/lindane/lindanefdaapproachchart.pdf>.

USA. U.S. Environmental Protection Agency. Pesticides. Lindane Voluntary Cancellation and RED Addendum Fact Sheet. July 2006. U.S. Environmental Protection Agency. 23 Dec. 2008 <http://www.epa.gov/oppsrrd1/REDs/factsheets/lindane_fs_addendum.htm>.

USA. U.S. Food and Drug Administration. Center for Drug Evaluation and Research. Lindane Shampoo and Lindane Lotion. 28 Mar. 2003. U.S Food and Drug Administration. 23 Dec. 2008 <http://www.fda.gov/cder/drug/infopage/lindane/default.htm>.

Washington, George. "The Rules of Civility and Decent Behaviour in Company and Conversation." Amy Ridenour's Historical Documents. The National Center for Public Policy Research. 23 Dec. 2008 <http://www.nationalcenter.org/WashingtonCivility.html>.

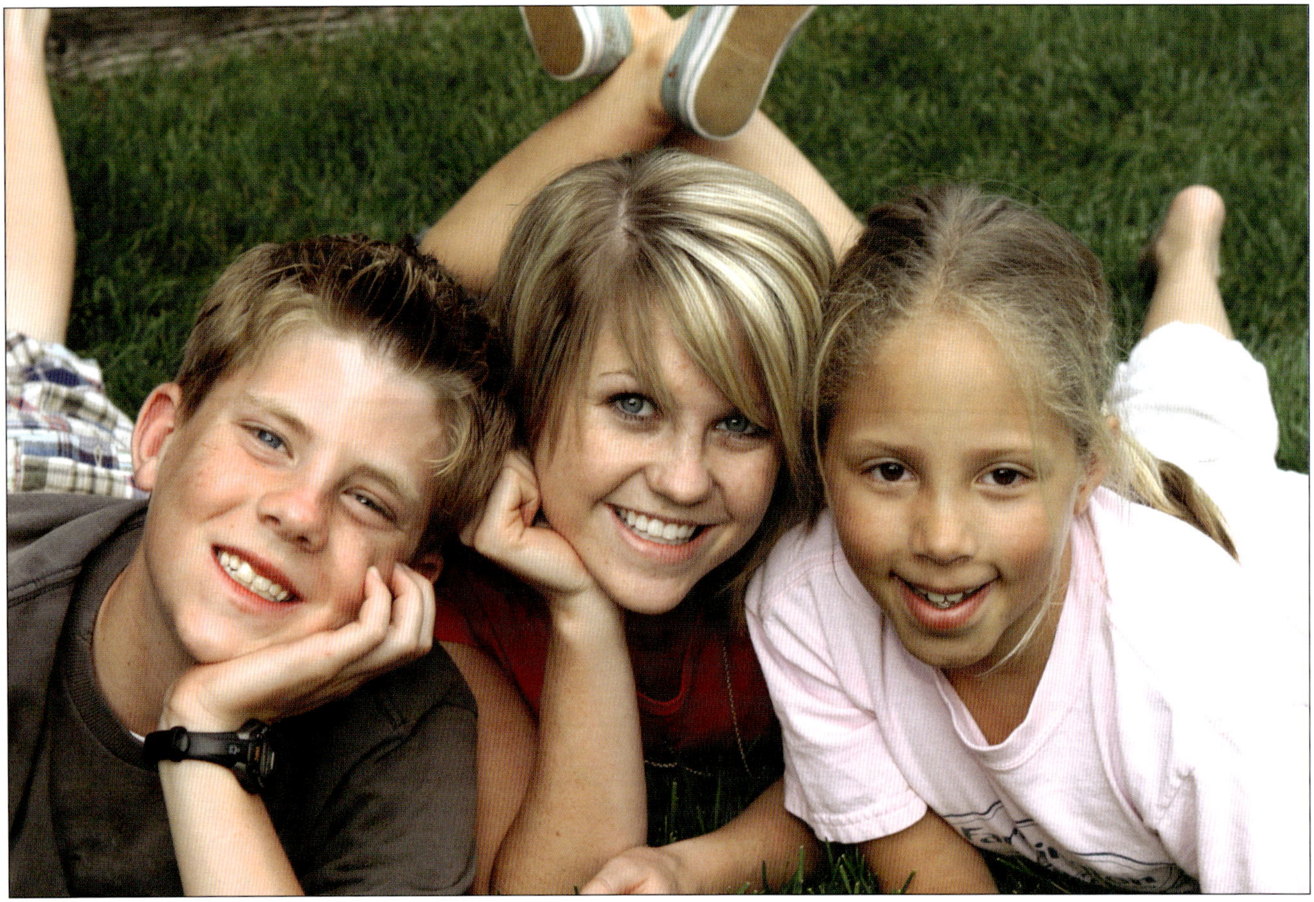

TESTIMONIALS

Before starting Fairy LiceMothers, we wanted to make sure we knew as much about lice as possible. We did a lot of research on our own and looked at a few other techniques for eliminating lice. I have to say that none compare to the effectiveness of the Shepherd Method. The information I have learned from Lice Solutions is invaluable. I feel totally confident in everything I tell my clients. Thank you Katie for the in-depth training and continued support Fairy LiceMothers receives from Lice Solutions.

Fairy LiceMothers – New York
888-561-0492
www.fairylicemothers.com

After battling head lice with my own children I knew that help had to be available for more parents. Determined to provide the best service possible I traveled to West Palm Beach, FL, where I participated in an intense training program. I was most impressed with Katie Shepherd's expertise and was excited to share her technique with parents in the San Francisco Bay area.
Thank you, Katie, for your continued support and for the help that you and your staff continue to provide to Lice Patrol. I strongly recommend this training to anyone who wants to learn about head lice.

Martina Mitchell
Lice Patrol – San Francisco Bay Area
www.licepatrol.org

As directors of a resident camp we feel strongly about maintaining a lice-free environment. Lice Solutions acts as our partner and an extension of our camp health center. The Lice Solutions staff screens our campers and staff at the beginning of each session, trains our health center staff in appropriate follow-up care, and educates our whole camp population. Our partners at Lice Solutions help us to continue to provide safe and memorable summer experiences to our campers.

Corey & Justin Dockswell Directors,
Camp Wicosuta, Hebron, NH

As a parent I am frustrated by the lack of safe products and the large amounts of inaccurate information regarding head lice. Katie, however, has the "hands-on knowledge" that sets her above the rest. When I talk to others about lice, I tell them to look no further; the bible of head lice is with Lice Solutions. Thanks to her valuable information, I was able to fight our public school and keep our head lice checks and no-nit policy in our school. Thank you, Katie, for being a mentor, advocate and educator to so many families throughout the US!

Kelly R. Addison,
Reeseville, WI

Katie Shepherd and Lice Solutions are THE experts in the field of head lice. She has worked tirelessly to educate the public and help all of those in need - regardless of their financial situation. Katie has served as my mentor for many years, helping me to perfect my company's lice removal technique and is a constant source of support. Katie has earned the respect of all in this very unusual field. My hat is off to her and for all she has done and will continue to do.

Penny Warner, BSN, RN, NE-BC
President/CEO
The Texas Lice Squad
www.texaslicesquad.com

Thank-you Lice Solutions!

You were there when we needed you. Despite my after hours call, you stayed late into the night to help my family so we could leave on vacation the next morning. We are so grateful to all the staff. You went above and beyond expectations, and we were able to leave for vacation on time and bug free!

Cathy Ferro
Palm Beach Gardens, Fl.

I just wanted to thank you for all the extra hand holding you did while I was in your office with my three children. Although it was an itchy experience for us both physically and mentally, it was great to have Lice Solutions to get us through it. I will suggest you to anyone that I know who needs lice services in the future. Thanks again!

Jamie Stevens
Lake Worth, FL

Katie Shepherd's Lice Advice book is a perfect tool for parents and school nurses. The Shepherd Method proves that lice control and prevention is possible using natural methods. Fairy Tales Hair Care is so pleased to offer this invaluable source to our customers.

Risa Barash, Owner,
FairyTales Hair Care for Children

Thank you for checking my entire family and assuring us that not all of us had lice and therefore not all of us needed to be treated. You made a bad experience better by just being there.

Kim Hurst
West Palm Beach, Fl.

Head lice infest millions of schoolchildren annually and can make any parent's skin crawl just thinking about the unwelcome guest that may accompany a child home from school. Clearing up the misconceptions surrounding this parasite with the latest information, Katie Shepherd's Lice Advice puts parents' minds at ease by clarifying why lice thrive and, most importantly, how to safely and effectively rid the nits from children's hair.

Jenna Greditor, editor of PARENTGUIDE

I am writing in support of Katie Shepherd's expertise and long experience in the field of battling head lice. Her method of combing out head lice is extremely effective. I have known Katie and worked with her now for several years. She and her staff are among the best in the business.

Dr. Dale Clayton
Professor of Biology
University of Utah and Founder & Chief
Scientific Officer, Larada Sciences, Inc.

I just want to thank the entire staff for helping my family. You all are truly wonderful and I appreciate being able to lean on you when I had no one else to turn to. I admire all that you and your organization do for our community. Much appreciation and thanks.

Sharon Robinson
Greenacres, FL

I sent a student to you yesterday and I wanted to let you know that the father was thrilled with the care that his daughter received from Lice Solutions. He was full of information and wanted to share that information. This is wonderful speaking from a school nurse perspective. He is planning on telling all of his daughter's friends' parents. Thank you!

S. Robbins, R.N.
School Nurse

My daughter had been infested and reinfested for months. We have tried various products to remove and to deter infestation, but yet they kept coming back. I tried to find the miracle product but it was Katie Shepherd that explained that the problem was more likely in the treatment. Thanks to her for taking the time to talk with me and explain where my focus needed to be. My daughter has been lice free for 8 months now and we can finally breathe easy. Parents in South Florida are lucky to have her service!

Tracy Burn
Bethesda, MD

Finding Lice Solutions and meeting Katie Shepherd when both my daughters had lice was a godsend. It was the first time we ever had a problem with lice, but I had feared it for years after hearing other mothers' stories. I was ready to burn down my house, but the genuinely professional care we received from the well-trained staff of Lice Solutions was truly remarkable. They calmed me down, took their time with us, did a completely thorough job and followed up with us in subsequent weeks. With the amount of hair my girls have, I don't think I could have treated them nearly as effectively as Lice Solutions. In speaking with Katie and her staff, I was very impressed with their knowledge of lice. Lice Solutions, a non-profit organization, is an asset to our community, families and schools.

Stephanie Cassatly
Jupiter, FL

Both my daughter and I have contracted head lice. I was able to do nit picking on my daughter, but I needed someone to check my own head. I can't tell you how much it meant to my daughter and I to have your service available. Although I thought I had done a good job on my daughter, I still had not got it all out. While flying to South Florida is not cheap it was worth the trip to know we are lice free! I am forever grateful!

Margaret Rapport
Philadelphia, PA

Head lice has proved to be a continuing challenge and Katie Shepherd has met this challenge. Not only did she meet the challenge, she has created a non-profit organization which educates, teaches, trains, and gives a wonderful non-toxic method for elimination. Learning about these parasites has given me knowledge which alleviates the fear of head lice and has also prompted me to begin my own successful business. Katie Shepherd's LS Training is forward thinking and successful.

Una Curran, owner
MOTHER'S HAIR RESCUE
San Francisco Bay Area
650-488-0238

The problem of head lice is growing across the world and resistance to pesticides is one of the contributors to this increase. As a business associate, I can honestly say Katie has impressed me as well as others with her persistence in educating the public about the nuisance of head lice. I have relied on her expertise to not only educate myself, but others as well.

Sherri Jones, CCRC, Project Manager

When I sat down with Katie on our first visit I will never forget how the staff greeted me and Katie showed me an understanding heart. She assured me that first and foremost, my daughter Sarah was very sweet and that was why the bugs loved her. I think I laughed through my tears as she further explained to me that it was Sarah's blood type the bugs were after, not her head of hair. This was the point at which Katie began to educate me and debunk the myths that so much of the general public walks around with. She took time out to really help us cope with our situation and provided us with several treatment options. I have always admired her devotion and patience.

The Dodsons-Dave, Barb, Derek and Sarah
Greenacres, FL

Katie Shepherd is to be congratulated on this new book which continues her dedicated efforts to eliminate the frustrations and potential risks of treating head lice infestations, a continuing cause of stress, anxiety and social stigma for millions of children and parents.

Nick Spring, CEO, Topaz Pharmaceuticals Inc.

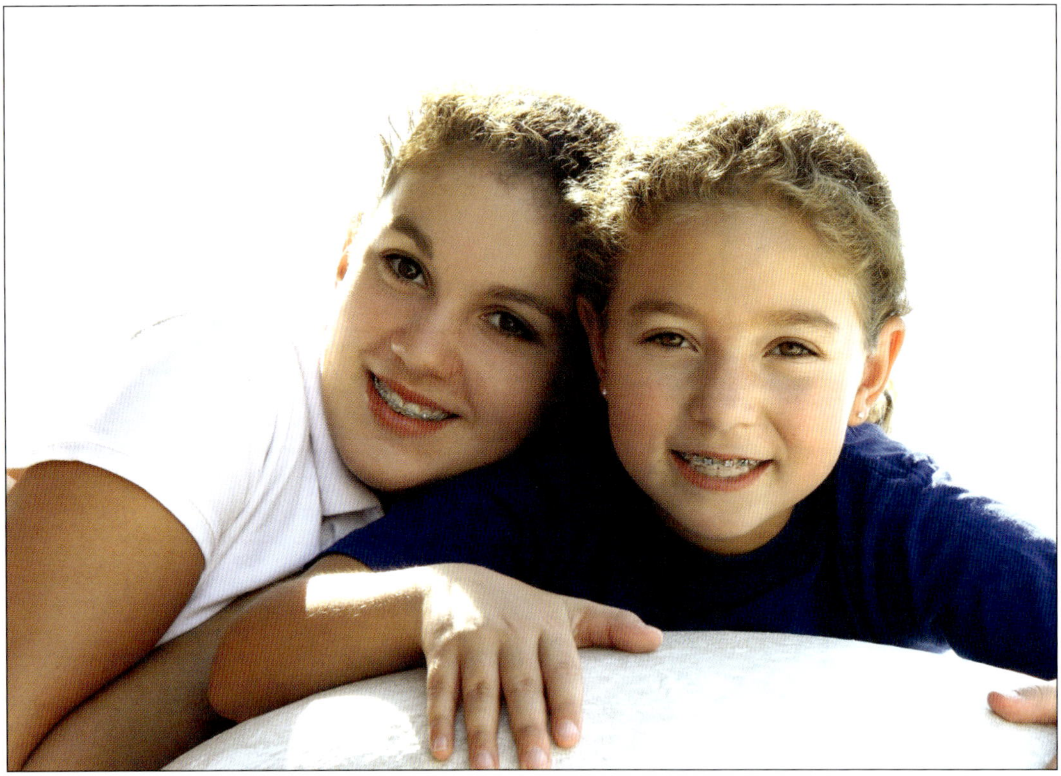

APPENDIX

For ease of use of this manual:

By placing tabs at key portions of this book, you will be able to move quickly through the various sections as you seek to eliminate your family's head lice infestation. While doing this is a personal choice, we suggest that you place tabs at the following pages with their corresponding headings.

Treatment facilities that are certified in The *Shepherd* Method™:

The following companies have completed a rigorous training program at The Shepherd Institute for Lice Solutions and have received certification in The *Shepherd* Method™ for treatment of head lice. We have listed them alphabetically by state and service. For the latest updated listing please visit the Lice Solutions website at www.licesolutions.org

California

Lice Patrol
San Francisco, CA
P. 415-566-LICE (5423)
www.licepatrol.org

Mother's Hair Rescue
San Francisco, CA
P. 650-488-0238

Florida

Lice Solutions Resource Network, Inc.
6758 N. Military Trail, Suite 110
West Palm Beach, FL 33407
P. 561-842-9969
www.licesolutions.org

The Nit Fairy
Tampa, FL
P. 813-376-5530
www.thenitfairy.com

Massachusetts

Nit B Gone
Boston, MA
P. 781-296-6201

New York

Fairy Lice Mothers
Oceanside, NY
P. 866-561-0492
www.fairylicemothers.com

Tennessee

Lice Solutions Resource Network, Inc.
604 Gallatin Avenue, Suite 105
Nashville, TN 37206
P. 615-227-3919
www.licesolutions.org/Nashville.html

Texas

The Texas Lice Squad
Pecan Plaza Shopping Center
2881 Dulles Ave.
Missouri City, TX 77459
P. 281-261-LICE (5423)
www.texaslicesquad.com

Information about the Terminator Comb™:

The Terminator Comb™ mentioned in this book is manufactured in Argentina and is marketed under various trademarked names. This comb can be purchased at www.licesolutions.org/comb.html in the US. The same comb is available in the following countries by these names:

USA & Canada	The Terminator Comb® or Nit Free®
UK	The Nit Free Nitty Gritty®
Australia & NZ	Nit Free Lice Breaker®
France & Spain	Assy®
Israel & Turkey	Assy®
Japan	Nit Free®
Latin America	Assy 2000®
Russia & Scandinavia	Assy®

Information about clinical trials for head lice:

Visit www.clinicaltrials.gov or http://clinicalstudies.info.nih.gov/ to search for current or to enroll in clinical trials for head lice.

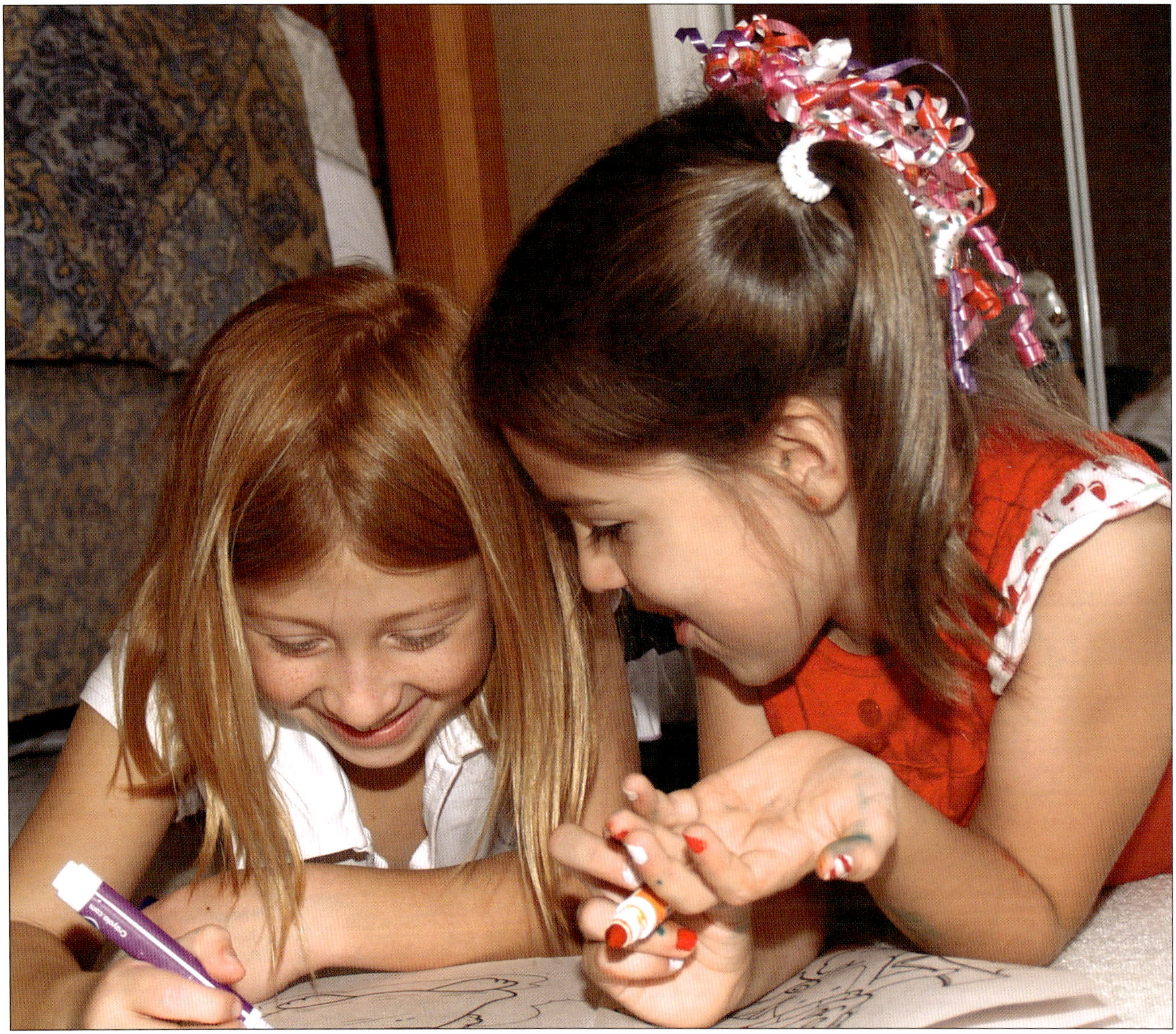

BIOGRAPHY

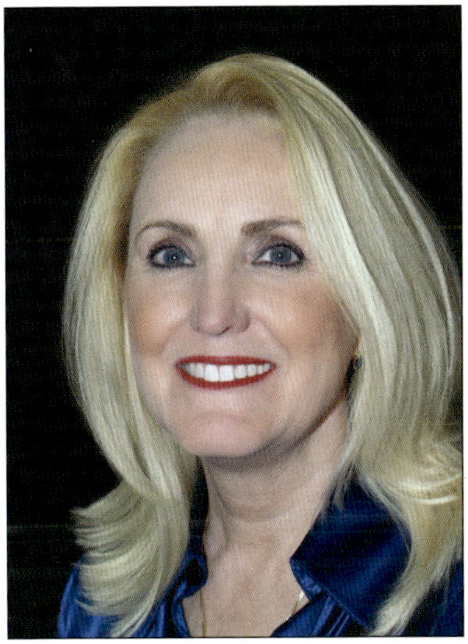

Katie Shepherd is the Founder and CEO of the Shepherd Institute for Lice Solutions in West Palm Beach, Florida. The Shepherd Institute provides ongoing training and certification for those seeking a career in lice removal as well as conducts clinical research in product testing and data collection. Ms. Shepherd is also Executive Director of Lice Solutions Resource Network Inc., a non-profit agency dedicated to reducing absenteeism through programs that provide safe and effective head lice treatments to school aged children and their families.

Ms. Shepherd's efforts address an issue few people want to talk about. Her inspiration came after she produced a segment called "The High Cost of Head Lice" for Kiplinger's Personal Finance Reports in 1997. Her research for this piece revealed that the problem of getting rid of lice was not so much product failures as much as treatment failures, and the lack of up-to-date lice information.

Determined to make a difference in her community, Ms. Shepherd organized an outreach program in 1998 that offered hands-on help designed to assist families in quickly eliminating the never-ending cycle of head lice. What started as a community outreach evolved into a non-profit organization that has helped parents around the world. With the addition of trained technicians and two offices, one in South Florida and one in Tennessee, Lice Solutions treats hundreds of families each week.

Recognized as one of the top lice experts in the industry, Ms. Shepherd has traveled around the world offering help where none was available. Thanks to her many ongoing collaborations with universities and researchers, Ms. Shepherd provides people with the most effective treatment options available and the most-up-to-date lice information in the industry.

As a mother of four and grandmother of five, she has devoted over ten years to helping make a difference in the lives of children everywhere. Ms. Shepherd lives in Jupiter, Florida with her husband Brad and daughter Ashley.

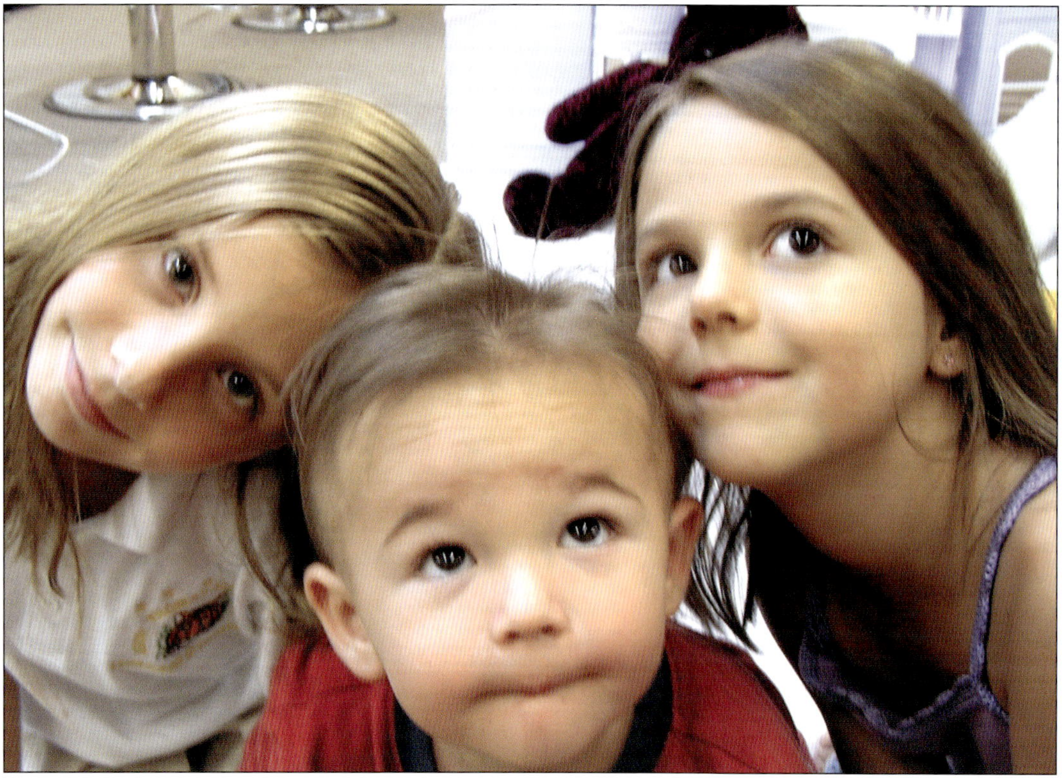

CONTACT INFORMATION

Katie Shepherd, Founder and CEO of The Shepherd Institute for Lice Solutions, devotes herself to helping families fight and win the battle against head lice through education and successful treatments. She has over 10 years' experience treating head lice and actively participates in research; partnering with several major universities, pharmaceuticals and product manufactures. She is Executive Director of Lice Solutions Resource Network, Inc. with the following locations:

6758 North Military Trail
Suite 110
West Palm Beach, FL 33407
P. 561-842-9969
F. 561-842-0311

604 Gallatin Avenue
Suite 105
Nashville, TN 37206
P. 615-227-3919
F. 615-227-3920

www.licesolutions.org

Information and services available through The Shepherd Institute for Lice Solutions include:

- Individual Treatments and Head Checks
- School-Wide Head Checks
- Summer Camp Programs
- Online Product Sales
- Group Presentations
- Intensive Hands-On Training & Certification Program in The *Shepherd* Method™ of Strand by Strand Nit Removal

Ms. Shepherd is available for speaking engagements, consultations, and training. Please contact her at the West Palm Beach, Florida office. To order additional copies of this book, visit: www.liceadvicebook.com

NOTES

NOTES

NOTES